Abby

Abby

✦

A Mother's Memoir of Losing One Daughter and Being Saved by Another

LESA KELLEY STEMBER

iUniverse, Inc.

New York Lincoln Shanghai

Abby
A Mother's Memoir of Losing One Daughter and Being Saved by Another

iUniverse books may be ordered through booksellers or by contacting:

iUniverse
2021 Pine Lake Road, Suite 100
Lincoln, NE 68512
www.iuniverse.com
1-800-Authors (1-800-288-4677)

ISBN-13: 978-0-595-40603-6 (pbk)
ISBN-13: 978-0-595-84969-7 (ebk)
ISBN-10: 0-595-40603-3 (pbk)
ISBN-10: 0-595-84969-5 (ebk)

Printed in the United States of America

For Jamie, Peyton and Tyler—my love for you defies words.
And for Abby, as I promised you…we will never forget.

Acknowledgments

First and foremost, I want to express my undying love and gratitude to my husband, Jamie, with whom I survived the journey told in these pages. Your unbelievable strength and love allowed me to live each day, and your continued support made this possible. You are my rock. I love you. And to my sweet Peyton, you truly saved my life and I hope that one day you know this. You and Tyler are a continued source of indescribable joy and love. I also want to thank everyone at Women's Healthcare Associates for their limitless compassion and tenderness, especially Terry DeFilipo whose gentle spirit and kindness were a constant source of strength. Thank you to my friends and family for their love and support during our loss of Abby, and your continued support as I embarked on the task of sharing what happened. And to Leslie, thank you for being my constant cheerleader in this undertaking and for always being there for me. I love you.

Introduction

The pages that follow contain almost every excruciating detail of the loss of our daughter, Abby. Please know that every word and experience are true and that my intent in sharing this with the world is to fulfill the promise I made to Abby to never let us forget her. Before each chapter, I have written a poem foreshadowing the chapter and giving further insight into the emotional turmoil of losing a child. I wish to allow you to see into the depths of this experience so should you encounter someone with a similar loss, you will hopefully understand.

The alchemy of my life, this pen.
With each stroke my spirit bleeds.
Yet, it is rejuvenated.
How powerful is watching my soul pour onto a sheet of paper through this ink.
I thank God for these words, for this expression.
If I were forced to hold this within my heart, my soul,
I would surely suffocate from its weight.
By simply putting this pen to this paper,
my soul and all of the pain and confusion in my heart are released through these infinitesimal drops of ink.
How soothing to lay my soul on a sheet of paper.
It need never be seen again.
Just to place it there, out of my spirit, out of my mind,
is to release its weight and breathe again.

1

No.

I stared at the pregnancy test. The faint line stared back at me. Hands shaking, heart pounding, I slid over to the kitchen window where the brutal August Florida sun burst through. I tilted the test into the light and focused intensely. The line seemed darker. Was it possible that somehow in the three seconds it took me to walk to the window that I had grown more pregnant? I continued to stare at the glowing line, thinking it might disappear. When it did not, I knew that I had to share with my husband, Jamie, the news of our third pregnancy in six months. In Prattville, Alabama, where I grew up, they had a name for women like me: "Fertile Myrtle." Jamie could simply glance my way and I became pregnant.

My problem was staying pregnant. Through tears, I convinced Jamie when our daughter, Peyton, was not quite two that she should not be an only child. I had images of a lonely childhood for her, with family vacations and no one to play with, tagging along after Mommy and Daddy to museums and fancy restaurants. Even in the fun places like Disney World, there would be no one who truly understood her incredible joy in meeting Cinderella or Ariel. I did not want that for my Peyton, the joy of my life and my reason for living. I wanted a childhood for her filled with bubble gum in her hair and a younger brother or sister who would torture her by repeating every word she said or cutting off the hair of her favorite doll.

I had accepted that I was pregnant with Peyton only after taking three home pregnancy tests and visiting my doctor for a blood test. The final test in hand, I had crept into our living room and announced, "Honey, I took three tests today and they were all positive."

Not turning from the television, Jamie absent-mindedly queried, "What kind of tests?"

When the truth settled into his brain, the shock was understandable. I learned we were pregnant with Peyton after only four-and-a-half months of marriage. A pilot, Jamie flew corporate jets for a charter company out of Fort Lauderdale. His arguably glamorous job kept him away from home most nights as he jetted celebrities all over the world, often spending weeks in exotic locations like Rome or the Caribbean. I could count on one hand the nights he slept at home during those first few months of our marriage. We teased that Peyton's conception was miraculous.

Being a pilot's wife required an enormous amount of patience, understanding, and independence. I often received calls on the nights Jamie was scheduled to return home that began with a hesitation, punctuated with a sigh, followed by, "Honey, there's been a change in the trip."

Three days would stretch to a week, then two. I quickly learned not to trust that he would return as scheduled. Some nights I happily came home after my day as a trial attorney making court appearances and taking depositions and collapsed into the couch with take-out and the remote. Other nights, I snuggled tightly with our two dogs, Paisley and Taylor, to ease the loneliness. When Jamie was hired by American Airlines when Peyton was only a few months old, normalcy replaced our erratic existence.

Now, with this fourth and most recent pregnancy, I needed to be sure. I quietly slipped into the bathroom while Jamie slept and rummaged the cabinet. Of course I had a stash of pregnancy tests. When you are "trying" you always have several around just in case you feel a little queasy or you're dying for a double espresso. I pulled another test from the value-pack box and grabbed one of the mouthwash cups under the sink. After filling it, I dipped the test with trembling hands. Rather than waiting the suggested three-minutes and praying, I watched the test. The faint line appeared immediately.

Whispering, I rehearsed my speech in the mirror. I considered, "Honey, I took a test and it was positive," but decided the sentence was too ambiguous. I thought I might try bluntness: "Honey, I'm pregnant." While to the point, it seemed a little too much for someone who needed fifteen minutes to wake up. Finally, I just walked into the room and somehow told him. Staring at me through bleary eyes, he simply croaked, "Okay."

My apprehension reflected my own fear, rather than his disbelief. In March, and then again in July, we had endured the heartache of two unexplained miscarriages. My pregnancy three years earlier with Peyton had been such an easy thing. Three positive tests, monthly visits, her perfect growth, and a painless birth under a blessed epidural at 39 weeks at exactly 7:00 p.m. to the most beautiful girl in the world. We thought it would be so easy after that. Instead, I lost two pregnancies in five months, both at exactly seven weeks. We never found out why. Now, only six weeks after our second miscarriage, I sat staring at a pregnancy test with two lines.

That afternoon, I called to make an appointment with my midwife, Terry. I had heard of her practice from a friend and, although apprehensive about seeing a midwife rather than an obstetrician, decided to give it a try. At my first appointment with her two years earlier for a routine annual exam, she spent an hour with me, taking my medical history and asking me what I had planned for the future. I left her office that day with a prescription for both birth control pills and prenatal vitamins. Patient, gentle, and possessing an unbelievable bedside manner, she had been the one to break the news of both of my miscarriages with those three awful letters "NFT," meaning "no fetal tones" or no heartbeat.

This morning, I dialed her office and the appointment desk answered, "What is the nature of the visit?"

I sucked in a breath, then stammered, "OB."

Just hearing the words tumble off of my tongue made my stomach hurt. Would this end with another early morning at West Boca Medical Center, hooked up to an I.V., being spoken to kindly and in soft tones by an anesthesiologist who would then wheel me into an operating room for a "D&C" to have a tiny, dead baby sucked out of my body? D&C. Two letters with unspeakable gravity. I didn't know if I could handle it again, but I had no choice.

A couple of days later, after cycling through every emotion imaginable, Jamie and I decided to share our news with his parents at our usual Sunday night dinner. Every Sunday night we had dinner with Jamie's parents, then left Peyton with them for the night. It always pinched my heart to leave her, but I knew it was important for both of us that I did.

On this Sunday, I waited until Jamie's Mom, Sue, and I sat alone on the floor in the room they had decorated for Peyton. Toys lined one wall and a big girl bed covered with Pooh Bear linens sat against another. The bed had no headboard or footboard, but it wasn't needed. Pooh Bears, which were Peyton's favorite, danced across the big bedspread. Jamie's parents spared no expense or detail in making her, their only grandchild, a room filled with her favorite things. Peyton sat next to us, fishing through a box of old costume jewelry, gleefully using us as her mannequins. She handed us bracelets, rings, and frilly hats, which we happily modeled for her as we caught up on the week's events and gossip.

After some time, I cautiously began, "Well, we have some news."

"Yes?" She anticipated the words, having heard them three times before.

"We're pregnant again." My voice sounded flat, betraying neither my excitement nor my fear.

"Really? Wow. Okay." With two fingers, she mimed a zipper across her mouth, "I won't say anything, but I'll keep my fingers crossed." She smiled meekly but without enthusiasm.

I continued, fishing for hope, excitement, something, "I see Terry in a couple of weeks. We should see a heartbeat."

She gently touched my arm, "Keep us posted. Can I tell Pop?" Pop was Jamie's Dad.

Surprised that she thought she needed to ask I assured her, "Of course. You can tell whomever you want."

Her eyes reflected a cautious optimism, "Okay. I'll tell Mike and Stacey, too. But I'll keep it quiet for now."

I understood her hesitation but missed the unadulterated glee of three years earlier when we told her that we were pregnant with Peyton. She literally came out of her chair, screaming and crying with joy. Now, after having endured the loss of two tiny grandchildren, she protectively refused to get excited until we knew "everything would be okay." The often-overlooked travesty of a miscarriage is that the innocence and pure joy of learning you are pregnant, and sharing that news, is gone. It is replaced with a stone in your heart that weighs down the joy with a sense of impending doom.

The next morning, I called my Dad. My two unmarried brothers had no children, making Peyton the only grandchild. I knew that Daddy wanted more grandchildren and that his heart had broken with our miscarriages. A devout Christian who believed strongly that life begins at conception, he sincerely mourned our losses.

I heard the smile in his voice, "Well, Baby, that's great."

He cautiously congratulated us and I promised to call with any news. As I hung up, I reflected on how wonderfully our relationship had evolved. My father had always treated me with respect and trusted my judgment, but since becoming an adult, he considered me a friend. I treasured this, his trust and confidence in me. I never felt as though he second-guessed or judged me. For this, and myriad other reasons, I adored him.

Telling my friends was a certainty. Many people wait to share the news of their pregnancies, especially in our circumstance, fearing something will go wrong and they will have to explain over and over again what happened, when they want nothing more than to forget. For me, enduring our miscarriages without our friends would have been impossible. I also felt that their knowing would make the tiny life hopefully growing inside of me more real.

Our best friends, Donnie, Leslie, Tye, and Kelly, planned to meet at Donnie and Leslie's for dinner a few days later. I decided not to tell them over the phone, even though I spoke to Leslie daily. She instinctively knew something was up, hearing the worry in my voice and knowing me so well, and kept asking if I needed to talk. I don't know why I couldn't share it with her yet. Probably for the same reason I couldn't get excited. I simply could not accept that I was going down this road again so soon. But my anxiety disappeared as we pulled into Donnie and Leslie's driveway. Despite everything that had happened, I could count on Leslie and Kelly to react as if nothing had happened, and, of course, they did. They both jumped up squealing and hugged me tightly. Genuine happiness replaced my apprehension and joy settled deep into my soul at last.

She steps through a billowy curtain blowing gently in the breeze.
So beautiful, so alive.
I immediately recognize her. Mom.
She reaches her hand out to me.
In her eyes, I can see that she is there.
There is no more confusion or emptiness.
I stretch out my hand to hers and as we touch,
my heart fills with her love.
That sweet, unconditional love that I have been aching to feel again.
The love that only a mother can give.
Her fingers are warm and I know that it is really her.
In that brief moment, my heart breaks with the heaviness of the aching I feel because I
miss her so.
I savor the love I see in her eyes,
because I know that it will soon be gone.
As will her memory.
I awaken and my heart breaks once again.

2

I had learned in the past six months not to go to the doctor too soon. Better to go when we expected a heartbeat around seven or eight weeks than to go too early only to see the six-week "rice grain," our hopes raised then smashed at the next appointment by the deafening silence of no heartbeat. So, after three weeks of decaffeinated coffee and no sushi, the day arrived. As I pulled into the parking lot of Terry's office, I took a deep breath, steadying myself. Sitting in my car in that parking lot, praying, had become too familiar a thing.

I finally let go of the steering wheel and made my way to the elevator. As I pushed the button for the third floor, my heart pounded so urgently that I could hear it. When the doors opened and I stepped into the waiting room, the sea of pregnant women overwhelmed me. I wanted to run back into the elevator, disappear out the front door, and pretend for a little while longer that everything was normal. Instead, I took a deep breath, summoned a hint of courage, and made my first steps toward this latest adventure.

When Terry greeted me her eyes twinkled, "I'm so happy to see you. So how far along do we think you are? Your D&C was just July 19th."

Sitting on the edge of the exam table, I kicked my legs back and forth like a child, then wrung my hands and strangely apologized, "Yeah. I know we should've waited a month or two after our last miscarriage. I must be more than seven weeks because I took the home test on August 24th and today's the 17th. It's my birthday, by the way."

"Happy Birthday!" Her voice filled with sincere optimism, "We should certainly be able to see the heartbeat on ultrasound. Let's take a peek."

As I lay back on the table, I closed my eyes and prayed. I savored the moment, clinging tightly to the fleeing hope that we would see a heartbeat. The certainty that it would not be there permeated my mind, poisoning my joy. But when Terry began the ultrasound, there it was. A strong, rhythmic, 140 beats a minute heartbeat. I laughed. Not only were we pregnant, we were actually going to have a baby.

Because of my history, Terry promised me that I could make appointments for as often as I "felt comfortable." Realizing that I could not come in every day, we decided on bi-weekly visits. She assured me that we could do unofficial ultrasounds at every visit to measure the baby's growth. To watch this tiny life inside of me and make certain that everything was okay. I then held my breath for six more weeks.

On Halloween, I picked my precious Peyton up from preschool. A fairy princess dressed in a beautiful gown, she carried a magic wand. Being a fairy princess did not excite her as much as my spreading glitter all over her face. I promised to take her trick or treating after my appointment with Terry.

Although the pregnancy had progressed beyond the seven-week mark at which I had lost my other babies, Halloween signified the pivotal day in my mind because the baby would be thirteen weeks. At the end of the first trimester, at thirteen weeks, my chances of having a miscarriage plummeted. I no longer would have to worry.

As we walked into the office, everyone made such a fuss over the little fairy princess holding my hand. When strangers reacted that way to Peyton, I always awed at the fact that this beautiful, sweet child was mine. I rested my other hand on my belly and said a quick prayer. While making our way to Terry's station, the nurses stopped and spoke to Peyton. They all had Halloween candy stashed in the pockets of their scrubs, which they freely offered to the beautiful fairy princess.

Moments later, climbing onto the exam table, I finally told Peyton that she was going to be a big sister. I explained that Ms. Terry would soon put a magic wand on my belly and let us see the baby inside. I no longer doubted. Terry squirted gel on me and began moving the ultrasound wand in slow strokes. I giggled when I saw the baby flipping around. The measurements confirmed that the baby was, in fact, thirteen weeks and growing perfectly. We saw little fingers and legs and a tiny little face. I again prayed, this time with a thankful heart.

We scheduled my next appointment for three weeks later, rather than two, because it would be time for my sixteen-week ultrasound. A technician would squirt more of the oh-so-cold gel onto my expanding belly and study the baby from head-to-toe. This would give Jamie and me not only the reassurance we needed, but we could learn the gender of our little miracle. Many people wait for the surprise at birth, but to me the surprise existed simply in finding out. I also refused to wait because, as a bit of a control freak, I needed to plan every little detail. When we brought Peyton home from the hospital, her clothes had been washed and put away, powder and baby lotion opened, and diapers stacked neatly under the changing table.

Three weeks later, the day finally arrived. With Jamie and Peyton beside me, we saw the baby's heart beating quickly. No matter how many times I saw it, I never grew tired of seeing that strong little heart beating furiously. We saw the spine, the legs, the arms, and even the fingers. All ten of them. The tech pointed everything out, assuring us it all looked fine. Then, we saw the eyes and nose, and the outline of a beautiful face. The baby sucked a thumb and appeared to be looking back at us. We caught a quick glimpse between the legs and learned we were having another little girl. I began to cry.

One week later, I hurriedly decorated our Christmas tree while preparing to go to Tallahassee for the weekend. Our neighbors, Bob and Pat, had given us tickets for the annual University of Florida-Florida State football game the Saturday after Thanksgiving. An FSU graduate and a die-hard fan, Jamie loved college football. He knew every player, statistic, and play. This kind of focus was both his greatest strength and his greatest weakness. He would do anything required of him, if explained to him in painstaking detail. Without a checklist, it just didn't get done. I called it "the pilot thing." Most of my girlfriends were also married to pilots and we joked about the need to give our men explicit instructions. The prodding was a necessity rather than nagging. So as I multitasked at packing, getting the house situated, and putting the Christmas tree together, my husband screamed at the television as he watched some obscure college football game gleefully.

Bob and Pat, who lived just two doors down, befriended us shortly after we moved into the neighborhood one year earlier. Jamie and I, early thirties with a two-year-old, became fast friends with this fifty-something couple that had been married for twenty-five years and whose two children had fur. I loved spending time with them. Pat and I had the most wonderful chats, speaking of politics, family, religion, and current events. Our conversations were fluid and intense. The youngest of four daughters raised in a traditional Catholic home, she surprised me with her progressiveness, having kept her maiden name and deciding not to have children. She and Bob adopted Peyton, stocking their home with chocolate sprinkles, Barbie DVD's, and Pooh dinnerware.

I had insisted that we put our Christmas tree together before leaving for Tallahassee because I wanted it up for the entire month of December. Growing up, Christmas was a magical time in my home. My Mom would decorate the tree with homemade ornaments while my brothers and I strung fresh popcorn. Although it was a certainty that I would stick myself several times, I loved this tradition because my Mom made us feel as though she needed us to do this for her. I now realize this ingeniously kept us occupied while she placed the ornaments on the tree just so.

Thinking of her, I fought back tears. For several years now, my beautiful 52-year-old Mother was slipping away as her frontal lobe dementia progressed. Similar to Alzheimer's, her unique dementia not only robbed her of her memories, but it robbed us of her spirit long before we were aware of its presence. She usually remembered my father and me, but her ability to comprehend was diminishing to the point that she was incapable of real conversation. At first, we didn't realize what was happening to her because her personality changed before any recognizable symptoms surfaced, and she was so young.

The first inexplicable slap-in-the-face occurred four years earlier when she phoned only two weeks before my wedding to tell me that she was not coming to Florida for the wedding. Through sobs, she explained that her back hurt and she didn't think that she could sit on a plane for two hours or stay in a hotel. Her words hurt immensely. I remembered thinking, "I'm her only daughter. Her first child to get married, and she isn't coming? She tells me this now? Two weeks before my wedding?"

I had wept bitter tears to Jamie, unable to believe that my own mother could not deal with a backache to come to our wedding. "It's not cancer! She isn't immobile." I had cried to him. "It's a backache. She doesn't even take pain pills for it. How bad can it be? She can't suck it up for a couple of days to watch her only daughter get married." To pass the time, she would sit for hours and cross-stitch beautiful designs, but she couldn't endure a two-hour plane ride? My wounded feelings succumbed to my anger.

That day solidified my certainty that Jamie was truly the one. Of course I'd had my suspicions, I *had* agreed to marry him, but that day, he demonstrated just how much he loved me, and just how wonderful he truly is.

"We'll charter a plane," he announced. "She can fly in that afternoon, be there for the pictures and the ceremony, and fly home. She won't be gone for more than a few hours."

I protested. A charter plane would cost thousands of dollars for only a few hours, and I was furious at her for not loving me enough to even try to come on her own. Why should we go out of our way? Why should we spend money to pander to her selfishness? This was my wedding! It was a backache!

"I can't afford it," I retorted, which was the absolute truth. My student loans from law school measured in the six figures and I put every penny I didn't use to live towards paying them off. I had no savings.

He relentlessly insisted, "Lesa, she's your mother. How can she not be in the pictures? How can she not see you get married? You will both regret this. Let me do this for you. Please, I love you. I want to." So he did.

As I now hung one of the ornaments she had sewn when I was just seven, it saddened me that this awful disease was continuing to shred her mind. I could not share with her what had happened to me. I could not talk with her about my fear and apprehension at once again being pregnant. I could not share my joy at having been given another chance to feel the unconditional, indescribable love that one can only feel for a child. I missed her so.

After finishing the tree and throwing some clothes in a bag, we hopped in the car and headed for Tallahassee. Jamie uncharacteristically bounced out of the house, thrilled to be going to the game. Especially since Bob had scored tickets on the 49-yard line. We would tailgate before the game, scream until we lost our voices, then sleep in the next morning. This was a luxury now that we had a two-year-old.

I made certain to throw my baby name book in the car. I had been hounding Jamie about naming the baby, but we had been unable to agree on anything. He liked names that started with a "J" like Jordan or Jillian. I liked beautiful names that dripped off my tongue and evoked images of fairies and tea parties: Emily, Emma, and Sarah. While outwardly appearing open to suggestions, I knew he had decided on his few. I admired how easy it was for him. I took choosing a name for the baby very seriously. This would be her identity and would always precede her. Although not of her choosing, her name would make an irrevocable first impression. I wanted a sweet name that reflected strength.

An hour into the eight-hour drive to Tallahassee, I pulled out the book. Jamie was trapped and I was determined. Realizing that the best way to handle this situation was to simply pick from his list, I told him to sound off all of the names that he liked and I would choose one. I proceeded to systematically dismiss each of his suggestions.

After over a dozen rejected names, he sighed, "What about Abby?"

I teased, "But honey, Abigail sounds like an old woman's name. Not the name of a little kid." I had two criteria: the name had to be cute when shortened, which was inevitable, and had to be appropriate for a young child.

"We don't have to name her Abigail if you don't like it. We can just name her Abby," he asserted.

I repeated the name over and over aloud, "Abby. Abby. Abby. I like it. Okay."

The decision made, our little miracle became Ms. Abby Stember, with her middle name to be decided. Her due date was May 10, 2003, just two days after my Mom's 55th birthday, which was strangely poetic.

They came for you,
the angels of death,
to steal you from me also.
But I scratched at them,
kicked at them,
drowned them with my tears.
Until they relented,
released their grasp,
and allowed you to fall into my soul.
Where you are safe.
In their absence,
I hear only the beating of your heart.

3

The entire town of Tallahassee buzzed. The intense Florida-Florida State rivalry fed the anticipation for their showdown, which was the final regular season game for both teams. We drove around town with Bob and Pat for hours, soaking up the electricity in the air, and ended up at Bill's Bookstore. Bill's served as both a necessity for students and the mecca of alumni seeking anything to catapult them back to simpler times. Funny how memorabilia can invoke feelings of youth, immortality, and sober intoxication.

We found an adorable little baseball cap embroidered with "Future Seminole" and bought it for Peyton. We poured over the adorable onesies searching for something for Abby, but nothing seemed quite right. My heart smiled as an image flashed in my mind. I pictured our girls and their Dad, trying to teach them the intricacies of football, completely unconcerned with their gender. By the time they started kindergarten, he would teach them the Seminole chant and how to yell "Go Noles!" After browsing around the store and tasting the excitement, we left for our hotel to rest before game time.

There are few things as exciting as being at a college football stadium in the South on rivalry game day. The parking lot was a sea of garnet and gold, and the smell of tailgating hung in the air. We drove our Expedition to a spot, pulled the tailgate down, and began the pregame eating frenzy of chips, dip, and all things bad for you. We watched as fans filled the parking lot, the noise growing louder. Unlike South Florida where we lived, Tallahassee had a temperate climate and as the sun disappeared, the air grew cool. We donned beanies and sweatshirts, savoring the crisp chill of the fall night. After our junk food gorging, we packed up and headed into the stadium in a parade of thousands. The excitement in the air was palpable.

The first quarter did not disappoint. The crowd responded to each second of the game, with the roar echoing off the immense stadium walls. We jumped from our seats and screamed at the team. The band blasted and thousands danced in unison. The thrill of it all was intoxicating. At the end of the first quarter, Jamie and I decided to head down for a bathroom break and some refreshments. He made his way to the food counter while I joined the endless snaking line to the ladies room. I smiled as I remembered, "Hey, I'm seventeen weeks today." Each week a milestone.

Moments later, after finally making it inside, I began crying uncontrollably. I saw blood. Not just a little spot or two, but a lot of blood. I shook my head, praying, "No, no, no, no. This isn't happening. No, this isn't happening."

Panicked, I ran to find Jamie. I grabbed his arm and he turned with a smile. When he saw my tear-streaked face, his eyes exploded with fear, "What's wrong? Are you okay? What's going on?"

"I'm bleeding," I whimpered.

He grabbed me and steered me out of line, "I'll go tell Bob and Pat we're leaving. I'm taking you to the hospital. Will you be okay here?"

I could barely speak, "Yes, baby, just please hurry. I'm so scared."

He touched my cheek, "I know. Just hold on."

As I stood at the bottom of the ramp, the tunnel blurred. The roar of the crowd and the announcer's voice became muffled, as if I were under water. Everything shifted in and out of focus and my head began spinning. I gasped for breath and grabbed the railing. Several people stopped to ask me if I was okay. I was crying so hysterically that no one who passed by ignored me, even though I felt like I was disappearing. I had a surreal, out-of-body experience as the reality of what was happening sunk in. I was having another miscarriage. I simply nodded when anyone asked, "Are you okay?"

Moments later, Jamie, Bob, and Pat came running down the ramp. I begged Bob and Pat to stay and watch the game. Despite the gravity of the situation, my Southern instinct of not wanting to impose my problems on anyone kicked in. I didn't want them sitting and worrying at the hospital after they had come all this way to see the game. Thankfully, they insisted on coming with us. As we stood in front of the stadium waiting for Jamie to bring the car around, I broke down in Pat's arms, unable to control my sobbing. She cradled my head, stroked my hair, and began to softly cry with me.

Jamie screeched around the corner and we climbed into the car. As he pulled away, he headed the wrong way down a one-way exit from the stadium. We quickly saw lights as a police officer pulled us over. After taking an eternity to get out of his car, the officer walked slowly up to our SUV and shined his flashlight directly into Jamie's eyes, searching for signs of intoxication. He then shined his light in the backseat, "Why are you driving down a one-way street in the wrong direction and speeding?"

Jamie shakily replied, "My pregnant wife is bleeding and I need to get her to the hospital."

He flashed the light at me, blinding me, and moved it to my belly, which was not readily apparent as pregnant under my sweatshirt. The officer glanced back at us suspiciously, then looked at my face again. Seeing the undeniable terror in my eyes, he let us go with a warning. Jamie drove quickly, but in the right direction, to the hospital.

When we arrived at the emergency room, we were told there was an obstetrics emergency room in a separate area of the hospital. We searched the hallways until we found it, drawn by the sound of the deafening, unsynchronized whooshing emanating from the fetal monitors connected to several very pregnant women. I broke down as I explained to the triage nurse that I was seventeen-weeks pregnant and bleeding. She calmly handed me a hospital gown and pointed to the bathroom. I obediently walked toward it, furious at her cavalier attitude at what was happening to my baby. I later realized that her calmness was not only necessary to prevent the total hysteria that could have easily erupted in an obstetrics emergency room, but also from many years of knowing that most of the time, everyone was okay. What appeared to mothers-to-be as life-threatening situations for our babies was usually nothing more than dehydration or a typical, easily-treatable problem.

After fumbling with the gown and giving up on actually figuring out how to tie the ridiculous number of strings configured in an incomprehensible pattern, I tucked the gown around me and looked in the mirror. My face was streaked with tears and mascara. The fear in my eyes had been replaced with defeat. It then occurred to me that the bleeding had stopped.

The nurse smiled understandingly at me and led me to a bed in the back corner of the room. She pulled out a Doppler, which was a hand-held machine that would allow us to hear Abby's heartbeat, if it was still there. I waited anxiously as she placed it on my belly, then began sobbing again as I heard that sweet little pounding. The nurse quickly hooked me up to a fetal monitor and tucked a warmed blanket around me. I closed my eyes and savored the sweet, reassuring whooshing that meant Abby was still alive. Jamie went to find Bob and Pat to let them know that we had not lost her.

The nurse told me that the doctor was on his way, but assured me that bleeding during pregnancy was not abnormal. Of course this made no sense to me. Why would I bleed unless something was wrong with either Abby or me? I lay back on the table and waited for Jamie. As I lay there, I listened to the nurses questioning the other women in the curtains around me. "So you're 33 weeks and having some cramping?" "You're 28 weeks and can't keep anything down." I couldn't help but think how lucky these women were. Even if there was a problem and their babies delivered, they would be okay. My sweet Abby was only seventeen weeks. No modern miracle of science could keep her alive if she were born now. I closed my eyes and tried to rest.

After an eternity, the doctor appeared, his hair tousled from napping in the on-call room. Coffee in one hand, he flipped through my chart with the other. I repeated what I had told the nurse and revealed my history of two miscarriages. At this, his face changed and he summoned an ultrasound machine, which quickly appeared. A gentle, insincere smile crossed his lips as he fiddled with the machine. After squirting gel on my belly, he searched. I could not help but sob uncontrollably again when I saw Abby sucking her thumb, seemingly content. The doctor checked every inch of her before assuring me that she was fine. He matter-of-factly repeated that bleeding was a common complaint during pregnancy. My mind refused to accept this ridiculous notion, but I was too relieved to challenge his assertion.

My relief faded when he said, "Although I'm certain everything is fine, I would like you to have a more thorough ultrasound by our radiologist just to make sure."

"But I thought you said she was okay."

He touched my arm, "She is. I just want the radiologist to double-check everything and take some measurements. I know we're backed up in radiology, so rather than sit around here all night, why don't you just come back in the morning?"

My stomach tightened. They needed another ultrasound, but we were supposed to just go back to our hotel and climb into bed and sleep like there was nothing wrong? We reluctantly agreed and I dressed. My arms and legs were so heavy. I did not realize that it was after midnight until we were told to be back at the hospital at seven and I glanced at a clock. I apologized to Jamie for his having to miss the game when everything was seemingly fine. He looked at me as if I had slapped him and reassured me that nothing was more important to him than his girls. After sweetly sliding on my shoes for me and tying them, he guided me to the door.

Back at the hotel, I climbed into bed exhausted, dreading the morning and the eight-hour drive home to South Florida. I tossed and turned, unable to sleep as the hours slowly passed. The doctor's need to have me evaluated again created doubts. If he was so certain there wasn't a problem, why did I need to be seen again by another doctor? I also could not wrap my brain around the notion that bleeding during pregnancy was somehow normal.

I finally fell asleep around four, only to have the alarm shatter my sleep at six. I plodded to the bathroom afraid of what I would find, only to be relieved by the absence of blood. However, what I saw in the mirror shocked me. My red, swollen eyes and puffy face rendered my reflection unrecognizable. Clearly the result of crying all night.

We arrived at the hospital and found our way to Radiology. Because they were expecting us, we were taken right in. My heart smiled as I watched Abby peacefully moving around, sucking her thumb and kicking. At seventeen weeks, the kicks were barely noticeable, but having been pregnant before, I was aware of them. I closed my eyes and focused on these tiny feet dancing inside of me. Each step was a reminder that Abby was still with us.

We stopped at a gas station just before leaving town. As Jamie filled the tank, I finally called our parents to let them know what had happened. Not wanting to worry them, we had not called until we were certain that Abby was okay. Their voices were remarkably free of concern, but I knew they were terrified and simply being strong for us. They, as all parents, lived and breathed the pains and joys of their children.

Jamie and I drove the eight hours home in virtual silence, exhausted from the mental anguish of the scare and the lack of sleep. I wanted Jamie to call in sick for his trip scheduled to leave Miami International Airport that night, but he could not.

The next day, Terry hugged me with genuine concern and listened as I gave her a blow-by-blow, including my disbelief at the "normalcy" of bleeding. She offered to do another ultrasound to ease my mind and I, of course, agreed. I never grew tired of seeing that sweet face staring back at me from the monitor.

"How are you *really* doing?" she asked. Keenly aware of how difficult and scary pregnancy was for someone who had endured miscarriages, she listened to me voice my fear. The fear that I had not wanted to express to Jamie. She listened with her uncanny ability to make you feel as though you were her only patient and that she had nothing else to do but listen to you.

As she walked me to the door, I turned to her, "You know, the ultrasounds have reassured me that the baby's fine. I think that I'm making myself crazy, coming in so often. Since I can feel her, why don't we wait the usual four weeks before my next appointment."

"Are you sure?" Her brow furrowed, then smoothed, "I think everything is just fine, too, but I don't want you worrying. You know I'm here for you and you can come in whenever you want. If four weeks is too long, you call me."

"I know, Terry, and thank you for that. I truly know that. It's just that I need some normalcy. I'm really making myself nuts here."

She touched my arm, "Whatever you want, but you call me with any concerns. You can come in whenever." Then she hugged me good-bye.

A few days later, we had the gang over for a barbeque. Leslie, Kelly, and I settled into our usual spot around our kitchen table, while the boys sat out on the patio talking airplanes. When we all got together, we never stayed as one group. The boys always migrated towards shop talk while the women discussed friends, family, and, my favorite, books.

I pulled out the Pottery Barn Kids catalog I had been studying for a week. After much deliberation, I had decided on the bedding with tiny pink flowers. I thought that if we painted the nursery a pale green, the pink would be lovely rather than cliché. I had marked my calendar to order the bedding on January 11th, two days after my next appointment with Terry. Although I was absolutely convinced that Abby was perfect, our experience in Tallahassee reigned me in ever so slightly. Leslie and Kelly, of course, supportively approved of the bedding and its obvious femininity. We then began picking out bedding for T. Cole Balding, Donnie and Leslie's yet-to-be conceived son. We all agreed that the moon and stars pattern would go perfectly in the room right next to their master bedroom, which was already taking shape as a nursery.

Donnie and Leslie had been happily married and the parents of three beautiful dogs for eleven years. They had married young in their early 20's and flown around the world as a pilot and flight attendant for American Airlines. Wildly devoted to their dogs, they had not seriously worked on having children without fur. But lately, the bug had been biting and whether they should go for it was a recurrent topic of conversation around our table. Kelly and I attempted at every turn to convince Leslie that they should do it. Donnie and Leslie were the kindest, most open-hearted and loving people we had ever known. The idea that they would not have children seemed ridiculous. Whenever Kelly and I smelled a weakness in Leslie's resolve, we hammered away.

Tye and Kelly, on the other hand, were the unmarried couple of the group. Their wedding in April, just a few weeks before Abby was due, was the other frequent topic of conversation. Surprisingly, Kelly focused on their impending marriage as much as she did on the wedding. I always found this incredibly mature and thoughtful. When most 20-something women became engaged, myself included, the actual wedding planning shadowed any considerable conversation regarding the marriage. Discussing dresses, flowers, colors, and food was infinitely more exciting than discussing merging checking accounts, in-laws, and the division of household labor. Kelly always surprised me like that. She was only a few years younger than me, but she had a sweet naivety. Leslie and I both considered her the little sister we never had. Interestingly, her fiancé, Tye, had the same relationship with Jamie and Donnie, with its predictable brotherly teasing. Each of us brought something to the group that made us all stronger just being together.

Because Tye and Donnie were both scheduled to fly on Christmas Eve, I invited Kelly and Leslie to join our family for Christmas dinner. As a child, my Mom always celebrated Christmas with unabashed joy. The tree donned her homemade ornaments and decorations filled our home. Everywhere we turned, there was another candle or wreath or holly bunch. She would bake endless amounts of cookies: chocolate chip, peanut butter, and "candy cane," as well as my favorite, red velvet cake with homemade cream cheese icing. She was truly amazing and loved every moment of it. Her sincere joy infected our home.

I don't know when everything began to change. I can't pinpoint the year she stopped enjoying Christmas. The year it all became a bother. We never noticed the subtle changes, convinced that she suffered from depression or chronic pain. Who could imagine that a beautiful, vibrant 40-something woman's mind was succumbing to dementia? "An unexplained spontaneous genetic mutation" I was later told. At the time, it was simply a mystery.

I was determined to recreate for Peyton the mystical Christmases Mom blessed us with during my childhood. My Dad graciously gave me the homemade ornaments when Mom no longer decorated a tree. I then bought the biggest Douglas fir I could find and burdened its branches with her work. I also assumed Mom's ritual of playing nothing but Christmas music in the car throughout the entire month of December. She had created my love of the season and I wanted to pass that legacy on to my children.

Two days before Christmas, my Dad drove the twelve hours from Alabama with Mom, planning to stay only a few days. Her dementia made unfamiliar places uncomfortable and Dad didn't think she could handle being away from home for long. When they arrived, she shocked me. Even though we had visited them only a few months before, she had changed drastically. That was, unfortunately, typical now. She no longer wore make-up and had her hair combed into a very short Pixie cut. When I was a child, she refused to leave home without make-up and her hair curled just so. I wondered if she remembered this, or even cared anymore.

On Christmas Eve, I buzzed around the house as everyone arrived. Harry Connick, Jr. and Nat King Cole looped in the C.D. player as our dogs stole proscuitto from the coffee table. The house filled with laughter and the smell of roasting turkey. When Leslie arrived, she presented gifts for the girls, which Peyton tore open immediately. She brought pajamas and sparkling body lotion for Ms. Pey, and a tiny Pooh for Abby. Peyton appropriately named him "teeny Pooh" and begged to "baby-sit" him until Abby was born. I hugged Leslie tightly, loving her even more for having hope in Abby.

The night did not disappoint my expectations of a traditional, family Christmas. We gorged ourselves and had coffee, then sat as a family around the tree and watched Peyton open her gifts. In that moment, I was reminded how she had altered my world forever. I cupped my hands under my belly and caressed Abby. I could not wait to meet her and finally hold her safely in my arms. To love her with every inch of my soul as I loved my Peyton.

Peyton,
My sweet girl.
You are the embodiment of everything in this life that is good and beautiful.
To be cherished.
Since you came into my life, I can no longer breathe without you.
You are such purity, such beauty.
Your eyes are filled with love, with hope.
With such simplistic joy.
In you, I see everything I hope to become.
So understanding, accepting.
My love for you defies words.
They cannot capture the boundless joy I feel when I hear you laugh.
And the wrenching pain I feel when I hear you cry.
My one wish for you, my darling,
is that you one day hold your own angel
and experience the profound love I feel for you.

4

The Sunday before my four-week appointment with Terry, Sue and I took Peyton to the circus. She loved animals and Sue had gotten the tickets as a special treat. She adored Peyton and loved showering her with surprises. Being a grandmother suited her well, and she glowed when she was around Peyton. Jamie's father, Ted, was similarly smitten. He showed such gentleness towards her and was ferociously protective. I cherished the relationship Peyton had with them and felt infinitely grateful to them for their boundless love.

Throughout the show, the music blared, growing in intensity and building to a crescendo with each act. Abby moved and kicked wildly. At twenty-two weeks, she was big enough for me to feel her every move. I placed my hand on my belly with each jump, kick, and roll. As I watched Peyton, I realized that my sense of certainty had returned and that I was no longer apprehensive. Peyton was going to have a sister.

She loved talking to Abby. In the mornings, I would stand in front of the bathroom mirror in my underwear as I got ready for the day. Peyton would put her face up to my big belly and say "Hi, Baby Abby, it's your big sister, Peyton."

She'd chat about the games they would play and the toys she intended to share with her little sister. She grew increasingly impatient, asking me daily, "Mommy, when is Baby Abby going to come out of your belly?"

I would kiss her face and reply, "Soon, baby, soon."

Although she was almost three, Peyton still slept in her crib. We had removed the front railing the year before, making the crib a toddler bed with a big girl blanket and pillow. With Abby's impending arrival, we knew we needed to transition Peyton out of it. Because her third birthday was only weeks away, we told her that she was getting a big girl bed for her birthday. The three of us went shopping together, and she jumped from bed to bed, squealing with excitement. She finally decided on a beautiful off-white bed with a matching dresser and mirror, accented with pastel buttons and swirls. The mirror angled down, allowing her to stand in front of it and see her entire reflection.

That night, after moving her crib and changing table into Abby's nursery, the three of us assembled everything and made her bed. She proudly handed Jamie the tools, then helped me fill the new pillowcase with her pillow. The project complete, Jamie and I stood in the doorway, staring at her. Amazed at how quickly time had passed.

Before we could ask her if Abby could use her crib, she suggested it to us, "Baby Abby can sleep in my crib now that I have a big girl bed."

"What a sweet idea," we told her, allowing her to own it.

Later at bedtime, we had a small setback. Since the time Peyton was only a few weeks old, I had rocked her to sleep in her rocker every night and sung "A Groovy Kind of Love." All of the parenting books advised against putting your child to bed asleep, insisting that you tuck them in awake to teach them to fall asleep on their own. I would later regret not having followed this acutely correct advice. I had not intentionally rebelled against it, but simply loved rocking Peyton to sleep every night with her little arms and legs folded into me and my arms wrapped snugly around her. Children are small for only so long. I had chosen "Groovy Kind of Love" as her lullaby because of its lyrics. Every time I sang it to her, it brought tears to my eyes. By the time she was two, she had heard the song so often that she knew the lyrics by heart. It would tickle me to hear her crooning the pop song to her Pooh Bear as she rocked him.

After tucking Peyton into her new, big girl bed, she could not go to sleep. She begged for her lullaby. I sat down beside her on the floor, leaned over her, and stroked her hair as I quietly sang in her ear. She seemed so small in that big bed.

Days later, Donnie came over to help Jamie assemble an armoire for my computer, which sat in Abby's nursery. When Peyton was seventeen-months-old, I ended my career as a trial attorney to take a job as a case law editor for a legal publishing company, telecommuting from our den. The ridiculous hours required by my profession as a lawyer had taken me away from my precious Peyton. I knew that I did not want to turn around and ten years have passed with my missing her childhood and not really knowing her. Being a practicing attorney simply did not allow me to raise my daughter. For me, that was unacceptable. Just as I reached my breaking point, Sue, who worked as a legal secretary, told me she had heard about the editor position. It was such a blessing. I worked entirely from home, which allowed me to both be with Peyton and use my education. The best of both worlds.

Our house had only two bedrooms and a den, which I used as my office. Rather than bunking the girls together in Peyton's room, we decided to transform the den into Abby's nursery. The armoire would contain my office and go in our bedroom. I had planned to then have Jamie paint the nursery a shade of pale green. The first step towards readying it for Abby.

Because the armoire was completely unassembled, Jamie and Donnie worked the entire afternoon piecing it together. As dinnertime approached, Donnie agreed to stay since Leslie was out of town on a trip. Jamie and I both loved spending time with him. He was bright, kind, and knew something about everything. His positive attitude was infectious and he kept Jamie from throwing the drill through the window in frustration.

As I ran out to the farmer's market to buy steaks for them, it occurred to me that I had not felt Abby move all afternoon. I searched my mind, trying to remember the last time I had felt her. I quickly dismissed any worry, picturing her curled up asleep, warm and snug inside of me. Her most active time was always at night anyway. Every night at ten, like clockwork, she began her gymnastics. I would lift my T-shirt and place Jamie's hand on my belly as Abby flipped and kicked, sometimes so hard that Jamie's hand jumped. When I would finally roll onto my side to sleep, she seemed to calm down, as if she knew that Mommy needed rest.

That night as Jamie and I lay in bed, the completed armoire sitting in the corner, I tried to wake Abby. I waited until Jamie was sleeping, not wanting to alarm him needlessly. I resolved to ask Terry at my appointment the next day how much movement I should expect. I just couldn't remember how often I had felt Peyton move at six months. Lying in the dark, I quietly pushed on my belly, hard, several times, begging her to move. Then, I felt her. I felt movement. When she stopped, I pushed again. She did not kick me, but I felt her rolling around. Relieved, I slept.

My heart ripped open.
My blood, my life, oozed from every corner of my soul.
The pain clawed from within.
Through my skin.
I clenched my arms,
squeezing,
trying to contain my sanity as it, too, scratched and tore through.
Until I exploded.
My body unable to contain the excruciating pain.
I feared I would die from its magnitude.
It was not so merciful.

5

I sat in the waiting room at 4:45 PM, anxiously awaiting my 4 o'clock appointment. The unrelenting queasiness in my stomach caused me to clench my teeth. I had not felt Abby kick all day, but when I pushed on her, I would feel her move. At almost twenty-three weeks, and after countless ultrasounds, I convinced myself that the stone in my stomach was nothing more than paranoia. God certainly would not be so cruel as to let Abby reach six months and then…I simply couldn't finish the thought. Instead, I turned my attention to Peyton as she fluttered around the room. My little ballerina in her pink tutu and pink tights danced in circles and practiced her plies.

Finally, Donna, Terry's nurse, called my name. She smiled at Peyton as we followed her down the hall, "Sorry we're so late today. Terry had some things pop up."

Forcing myself to sound bored, I replied, "No problem. She never makes me wait. I figured something was up."

She turned to me, "How are you feeling?" Everyone in the office showed such empathy for what we had endured.

"Fine," I lied.

When Terry entered the exam room, she asked her typical, "Is there anything unusual going on or that you're feeling?"

"No," I quickly replied, but, then I reconsidered. "You know, she hasn't been moving very much in the last day or so. I'm sure I'm just paranoid. I just thought I would mention it."

She gently placed her hand on my leg, "I'm sure everything is fine, so let's take a quick listen to reassure you."

I lay back on the table and waited anxiously as she moved the Doppler across my belly, searching for a heartbeat. I scanned her eyes for reassurance. Instead, a look of worry slowly spread across her face, "You know, I'm not hearing anything, but sometimes it's hard to get a good read with this thing. Let's do a quick ultrasound. I'm sure everything's fine."

She grabbed my chart from the table and led me through the familiar maze of hallways until we reached the ultrasound room, which was occupied despite the late hour. I took Peyton's hand and led her to the seats that lined the wall opposite the room. The sick feeling in my stomach intensified and I fought hard not to cry. I was determined not to lose it in front of Peyton. My mind raced and I prayed frantically, "No, God, please don't let this be happening. Please, please, please, don't let this be happening. Please don't take Abby. Please let her stay with us. Oh, God, this isn't happening again. You wouldn't do this to us. Please. I felt her move this morning."

Then, it hit me. In the past few days, Abby had not flipped and kicked. Her movements had been slow and gentle. She had not responded to me. The movements were created by the momentum of her body. Momentum created by me. I grabbed my mouth. I was going to throw up.

The door of the ultrasound room opened and a couple emerged smiling and holding printouts, pointing at their baby. I looked down, unable to witness their joy. I did not want to poison it, even slightly, with the obvious pain in my eyes. Terry reappeared and ushered me into the room.

As I lay down on the table, the air in the room grew heavy. Terry attempted a stilted smile, but I could see it in her eyes. She knew something was terribly wrong. Without speaking, she spread the gel on my belly and slowly began moving the wand. Although the silence was immediately obvious, it took several seconds for me to understand. Abby's heart was not beating.

Baffled, I looked at her, "Why can't we see her heart beating?" In my mind, this was simply a technical problem. A machine malfunction. She needed to reposition me or something.

Terry turned her face from the monitor to meet my gaze. In her eyes, I saw sadness. She simply said, "I'm so sorry. There's no heartbeat."

My mind refused to accept the meaning of her words, "What do you mean? Where is it? Why can't we see it?" As if it were there, but undetectable for some reason.

"Lesa, I'm so sorry. The baby has died."

My stomach flipped and the room began to spin. A primal scream from the depths of my soul crawled up my throat. It froze when Peyton climbed onto the table, "What's wrong, Mommy? Why are you crying?"

Shocked back to consciousness, I knew that if I allowed myself to fully comprehend what was happening I would frighten Peyton. Even at this, the most horrific moment of my life, my thoughts were of her. I didn't want her to be afraid. I didn't want her to ever feel, for one moment, that she was alone. If I gave into the horror, I would collapse and she would be alone with strangers. I could not leave her. I had to hold it together. I refused to accept the news.

Terry gently placed the wand on the edge of the machine, "Lesa, I need to go speak with Dr. Arcelin. I need an OB to concur. Will you be okay in here for a few minutes?"

I could only nod.

After Terry left, I began shaking violently. My body refused to contain the hysteria flooding my mind. I kicked it away, fighting it off as it threatened to consume me. I stared into Peyton's bright eyes, clutching my fleeing sanity. She smiled, jumped off the table, and climbed into the chair next to me. I reached out my hand to her, gripping her tiny fingers, squeezing her little hand.

Moments later, Dr. Arcelin knocked on the door, and then slowly opened it, "Hi. I'm so sorry but I need to take another look. Would that be okay?"

With surprising calmness, I replied, "Of course."

I thought, maybe her heart had started beating again. In those moments after Terry left the room, I had prayed harder than I had ever prayed in my life. I remembered hearing stories of people who had cancer that just disappeared, or people who had died and seen "the light," only to come back. They credited the power of prayer. Maybe God had heard my begging pleas. Maybe Abby's heart was beating again. Maybe this was all a nightmare, or a miracle.

Within seconds, Dr. Arcelin solemnly repeated, "I'm sorry. There is no heartbeat. Will you come back to my office so we can talk?"

I stared at the monitor. My beautiful Abby lay peacefully. Her heart still. How could this be happening? I was almost twenty-three weeks. She was perfect. No deformities they had told us. No abnormalities they had assured us. She had ten fingers, ten toes, a perfect heart, a perfect brain. She couldn't just be dead. Perfect babies don't just die. This was crazy. This was not happening.

I gripped Peyton's hand as we walked to Dr. Arcelin's office. Terry appeared and placed her arm around me, guiding me, "Where's Jamie? Can I call him for you, or do you want to call him?"

My mind slowly remembered that he was heading to Miami to work, "He's headed to Miami. You should call his cell phone."

"Do you want to speak to him?"

"No." I feared that my telling him would somehow make it true. I could not let those words pass my lips for fear that my uttering them would give them power and truth. My heart ached for him. I pictured him sitting in his car in rush hour traffic in Miami, fighting his way to the airport, only to answer the phone and hear Terry's voice. He would sit in his car, in traffic, alone. Her words would hit him in the stomach and take his breath. I hated that he was alone and had no one to hold him as he felt the wave of anger and grief that would surely overcome him. He would then have to claw his way back up I-95, alone, and continue fighting traffic for another hour before reaching us. I wished to be with him in that car, in that traffic.

I called after her, "Terry?"

Her voice full of her own sadness, "Yes, sweetie?"

I trembled, "Would you call my mother-in-law? I need someone here to help me with Peyton. Please."

"Of course." She jotted down the number. "Is there anyone else?"

"No."

I turned to Dr. Arcelin who sat quietly at his desk with his hands crossed in front of him. He raised his head solemnly and looked at me sympathetically. His face reflected the sensitivity he had learned practicing obstetrics. He had certainly explained to countless mothers that their babies were dead.

His words slowly spilled into my brain, "Because you are beyond twenty weeks, we can't do a D&C. You have to deliver the baby. What you have to decide is when you would like to do that. There's no need to rush to make a decision. You can go home and rest and then go to the hospital tomorrow morning if you'd like."

"Can I go tonight?"

He hesitated before answering, "If you would like, but you may want to speak to your husband first."

"No. I want to go tonight." The decision came without deliberation. I believed in miracles and I knew that when we got to the hospital, her heart would be beating again. But if it was true, and she was gone, I couldn't stand the thought of having her body floating around inside of me. Dead. A chill raced through my body. I began to cry again. I could not stop the tears. I closed my eyes, begging them to stop.

A little hand touched mine. "Mommy, what's wrong?"

Before I could answer, Peyton's favorite nurse, Lisette, stuck her head in the door. She loved Peyton and always sought out little treats to give her when we came for visits. Seeing my face, she asked, "What's wrong with you? You okay?"

Without thought, I blurted, "I lost my baby." I could not comprehend the words spattering from my own mouth. My resolve to be strong for Peyton quickly failed as the weight of what was happening crushed me.

She gasped, "Oh, I'm so sorry. Is there anything I can do for you?"

"Yes. Would you please take Peyton? I need…"

She squatted down, hugging Peyton, "Of course. Come on, Beautiful, let's go see if we can find where the lollipops are stashed."

Peyton happily skipped away, "Be right back, Mommy."

Dr. Arcelin apologized again and left the room. Grateful for the solitude, I rested my head in my hands. As his words sunk into my bones, my mind spiraled out of control. I began to strangle on my grief. My heart fell and I thought I was fainting. My sobs grew heavy and my body began to ache. No matter how hard I cried, I felt no relief. A scorching pain shot through my eye as a migraine set in. My entire body rebelled.

Terry returned and closed the door, "I caught Jamie in traffic on 95. He's turning around and is on his way, but it will be a little while. I also got in touch with your mother-in-law and she is on her way, too. Where can I take you? Would you like to go to my office? What can I do for you?"

Her gentle manner soothed me. I forced a smile, "Nothing, thank you. Lisette took Peyton so I could catch my breath. Terry, I don't understand. She's so perfect. How could this be happening?"

She said nothing and took me in her arms and held me as I surrendered to my grief.

Because it was after six, the waiting room was empty. Terry led me to a chair and offered me a drink and a box of tissues. Peyton played nearby, hopping from chair to chair and singing. Her joy a strange contrast to the immense sorrow.

"Thank you, Terry, for everything. I don't need anything else. You don't have to sit out here with me. I know you have stuff to do."

She placed her hand on my leg, "I have nothing to do but sit here with you. I will wait with you until Jamie gets here."

And so we waited. The mind has such an interesting way of protecting us. When things become too overwhelming, it simply shuts down. As we sat, I was not sad or angry or confused. I was just there, kissing Peyton when she ran over to me, and watching her quietly as she played.

Suddenly, Sue and Mike, Jamie's brother, appeared. "Hi," was all I could say.

I saw the pain in Sue's eyes and she hugged me tightly. Mike quickly hugged me, too, with a confused, anguished look on his face. As I would quickly learn, people don't know what to say when someone loses a baby. The death of the elderly is expected. The death of a child, a baby, violates nature and baffles the human spirit. I thanked them both for coming so quickly.

"I'm going straight to the hospital. I'm too far along. I have to deliver her." The words sounded so clinical and matter-of-fact.

My mind continued to protect me from the absolute horror of the moment, "Would you please take Peyton home? Stay with her tonight? I don't know how long we'll be?" As if somehow we might be home by midnight.

"Of course," she whispered. "Whatever you need, I'm here for you. Pop, too. Just let us know what you need."

She then sat with me as I waited for Jamie. We agreed that she would take our SUV and Peyton home. Jamie and I would go to the hospital in his car. We sat quietly, solemnly, watching Peyton play.

I pulled out my cell phone, opened it, and mindlessly ran my finger over the numbers. I desperately needed to call Leslie. Not only was she my best friend, but she had an indefinable quality that relaxed me. No matter how stressful the situation, just being with her calmed me. I needed her. I knew that she would put aside her own pain over this and be there for me. She would be exactly what I would need her to be.

As my finger typed her number, I stopped myself. What was I doing? I could not do this to her. Jamie would be there. I wouldn't be alone. I desperately needed her friendship, but hesitated. I knew that if I asked, she would come. If I loved her, how could I force her to endure this? If she witnessed Abby's birth, saw her body emerge from mine…still…lifeless. I could not force her to endure that. Her memory seared with the image of my lifeless baby lying on a cold, sterile hospital bed. As much as I wanted and needed her there, I could not do that to her. I closed my phone.

After what seemed an eternity, Jamie walked through the door. I wanted to run to him, to fall into his arms and dissolve, but I couldn't. My legs refused to move. I saw the pain and disbelief in his eyes.

"I'm not going to hug you," Sue said quickly. We were all trying to be strong for Peyton, who continued to play, completely unaware of the horror around her.

Terry immediately reappeared, "Everything is ready for you. I've called ahead to West Boca, so they're expecting you. I'll check in on you in the morning, but if you need me before then, just let them know." She walked over to me and embraced me, "You know that I am here for you."

I nodded.

Peyton, thrilled at the surprise of Grammy coming home with her for a slee-pover, jumped into Jamie's arms. He explained to her that we were going somewhere else first, but would see her later. I took her from him, needing to hold her, and carried her out. As I placed her in her car seat, fear overwhelmed me. Suddenly, the thought of not being with her frightened me. I could not let her go out of fear that I would never see her again. She would not be safe without me. Recognizing the necessity of letting her go for now, I kissed her and closed the door. As they drove away, my heart collapsed.

The waves cover my head.
I stretch my arms to Heaven,
furiously clutching the air,
struggling,
fighting to live.
A force pulls me down,
under the water where I can't breathe.
Relentlessly, it pounds me.
Pulling me down.
Until I surrender.

6

When we arrived at the hospital, the triage nurse asked us to be seated because of the shift change. Our lives, our tragedy, were paused for this seeming mediocrity. Of course, the shift must change, but must we sit, twitching, in the lobby? Weren't we entitled to some special consideration? Apparently not. So we sat and waited with women whose swollen bellies could no longer hold their babies. Their living, kicking babies were forcing their way out. I moved to a side hall, unable to endure watching these women hold their bellies, panting as they paced impatiently as we all waited for the shift to change.

I went into the waiting room bathroom to catch my breath. Looking in the mirror, I frantically prayed, "Please let her kick me. Please let this be some mistake. Show me just how miraculous You are."

I was furious with God. He had taken two babies from me. He was slowly taking my Mom from me. Now, He had taken Abby, too. One tragedy per family, please. My prayer became frenzied, "What have I done to deserve this? Why are You doing this to us? Why would You do this to Peyton? Why would You take Abby? Why didn't You take her sooner like You took the others, instead of letting us get to know her?"

The excruciating pain in my head intensified with my defiance. I stared at the mirror, into my eyes, and saw such sadness and anger. Hearing no response to my pleas, I bowed my head and turned to the door. I took a deep breath and slowly pushed it open, guarding my eyes from the light. I found a chair in the side hall and cradled my head in my hands.

A nurse finally appeared and ushered us to my room. It resembled a bedroom with its flowery drapes, feminine bedspread, and television armoire. The only thing hospital-like was the warming incubator next to the bed, which was stocked with blankets, ready to embrace a healthy, screaming baby. Mercifully, the nurse quickly removed it, pushing it out into the hall.

After slipping into bed, I told her that I couldn't think or see. My head was exploding. She assured me she would get something for me after certain necessary questions.

"How old are you?"

"32."

"How many pregnancies?"

"Four."

"Live births?"

"One."

She stopped, "Listen, I'm the charge nurse tonight and I am going to take care of you. Dr. Arcelin prescribed Cervidil to induce your labor. It's just a small pill that I'll place in your cervix to cause contractions and dilation. Hopefully, we won't need to use Pitocin. I need to draw labs, but I'll do that when I do your I.V. After I get you settled, I'll bring you something for your head. Okay?"

I could only stare, certain my head would burst before she did what she needed to do. "Please hurry," I whispered.

As she left the room, I wanted to scream after her, "Wait! Aren't you going to do another ultrasound to be sure? What if they were wrong? What if she isn't dead? What if she came back to me? Shouldn't we be sure?" My lips betrayed me. They refused to move.

After she left, Jamie called his brother, Mike. Jamie was still in his pilot's uniform and needed clothes and food. They spoke briefly, only uttering what was necessary. Then, the two of us sat, waiting and staring at one another, not knowing what to say. My mind kept trying to comprehend what was happening. Unable to do so, it pounded. The rhythmic pulsing blocked out everything as I heard my heart beating in my ears. I asked Jamie to call my Dad, apologizing for having to ask. My sweet, strong husband simply agreed without question. Then, without my asking, he left the room to make the call.

A few minutes later, he returned, "He wants to come tonight. He says that they'll get in the car and he'll drive through."

I thought of my Mom. She had progressed to the point in her dementia where strange places made her uncomfortable. She would repeat, "I want to go home" over and over. I needed my Dad, but I could not handle being with my Mom and being confronted with another monumental loss. I could not watch her nervously fidget in her discomfort, insecurity, and fear. This would be difficult enough.

I held my head, squeezing it and scraping my fingers through my hair. Tearing at my scalp, I looked up with closed eyes, "Tell him, no. We don't know how long this will take, and I don't want to subject her to being here. If he can't leave her in Alabama, then tell him to wait until we're home."

Jamie paused, hating to insist, "Lesa, he really wants to be here."

I clenched my teeth and pain shot through my eye, "I know, honey, but I can't deal with my Mom right now. It's too hard."

My Dad agreed to wait, but only for a day. He told Jamie they would leave Alabama the next morning so they would be there when we went home. I took the phone. I could hear in his voice that his heart was breaking. I imagined how helpless he felt and how much he wanted to be with us. I wanted him there, too, but I just couldn't. It hurt to tell him no.

The nurse finally returned. She drew blood, inserted the I.V., and quickly showed me the Cervidil. Then came the Demerol.

As she slowly pushed the syringe, she spoke softly. Her voice empathetic and knowing, "Dr. Arcelin said that you can have Demerol every four hours if you want. Your contractions probably won't start for a while, but if you need to be less than lucid, I'll keep giving it to you."

"Please," I muttered.

She lifted my I.V. tubing and I felt warmth. Within seconds, I was numb and sleepy.

"Thank you," I whispered. I looked at Jamie, pained that he could not also be numbed. Then we sat, holding hands, as I drifted off to sleep.

Born in the face of death.
Each of us,
Born dying.
Yet it is not our own death we fear.
It is the death of those we love,
without whom we feel we will surely die.
That is the danger of love.
The danger of giving one's heart to another.
With a child,
there is no choice.
My heart was not given,
It was taken.
No manner of strength or will could have kept me from falling in love with you,
My Abby.
To give birth to you in death will surely kill my soul.

7

The next morning, Terry poked her head in the door around 8 while making rounds. My eyes, heavy from the many doses of Demerol, refused to cooperate. I glanced over and saw Jamie asleep in the chair next to me.

Terry tiptoed in, "I didn't want to wake you. I was just wondering how you were doing."

I smiled through closed lids, "Okay. The Demerol…"

"I know. Just try to sleep. If you need me, please just tell them to call me. I'm here for you. You know that. I have to go into the office, but I will be back later, okay? Dr. Rudolph is on-call today. She's wonderful, so don't worry."

I attempted a smile, then succumbed to the Demerol again.

A couple of hours later, an intense pain jolted me awake.

Jamie jumped, "Are you okay?"

I grabbed the sheet as the pain shocked me again. "Oh my God. Honey, please get the nurse. This hurts so bad. What is happening?"

Panicked, he raced to the nurses' station. The pain intensified. It was a burning, ripping pain that was tearing me in two.

Minutes later, a nurse, not my charge nurse, walked in. She matter-of-factly checked my I.V. bag, then asked, "Would you like an epidural? Are you in a lot of pain?"

I glared at her, wild-eyed, full of anger. In pain? Was she kidding?

As another pain scorched me from the outside in, I heard her repeat, "Epidural?"

My anger gave way to my desperation, "Yes, please. As soon as you can."

I wrenched as another pain shot through my body. I was being torn down the middle. I grabbed the side rails of the bed and began rocking back and forth, moaning. The sounds were primal as the pain was more intense than anything I had ever felt. Jamie paced the room, panic and fear in his eyes. I knew he felt helpless and afraid. I wanted to comfort him, but the pain grew more and more intense. The contractions drew closer together. He ran out of the room yelling, "Where is the anesthesiologist?"

A few moments later, the nurse returned with a syringe and announced, "The anesthesiologist is very busy. He isn't going to get here in time to give you an epidural. You'll have to do this without one. Would you like another shot of Demerol?"

"Yes!" I screamed. I would later regret taking the shot. With the many other doses, it left me completely dazed.

She inserted the syringe into my I.V. and I felt the now-familiar warmth, but the pain was so intense that the drug seemed to have no effect. I continued to writhe around the bed, watching helplessly as the minutes slowly ticked by.

The contractions came every minute, and lasted for most of them. There was no relief until I suddenly felt the urge to push. I began to cry uncontrollably. I wasn't ready. I wasn't ready to push her out. I wasn't ready to have her leave me just yet. I had rushed into this, deciding to come straight to the hospital. I needed more time with her, warm and safe inside of me. Once she was out, she would be gone forever. I sat up hard, fighting against the urge to push until it overwhelmed me and I could no longer control my body.

Jamie again ran for the nurse. She called for Dr. Rudolph, but there wasn't time. My body took over, ignoring the pleas of my heart for more time. At 10:26 a.m., after only three pushes, Abby's body fell to the bed. I could not look. I turned to Jamie, whose eyes were fixed at the end of the bed. His face was unrecognizable, morphed by what he saw. The room was excruciatingly silent. A single tear fell down his face, then another. It was the first time in the six years I had known him that I saw him cry. He didn't turn away from her. He kept staring at her, then whispered, "So pitiful."

Dr. Rudolph came running in. After checking to see that I was okay, she went to Abby. She removed the warm cocoon of Abby's amniotic sac and slowly wrapped her in a blanket. No one spoke. I turned my face away. The pain in my heart engulfed the pain in my body.

Then, Dr. Rudolph came to us, but I could not look at her, "We have to take her to the nursery to do some things. When you're ready to see her, just call the nurse and she will bring her to you if you want to see her."

As she turned and walked out of the room with Abby, I closed my eyes. My heart was empty and broken. The Demerol once again overcame my consciousness and I melted into the bed.

I pick up the broken pieces of my shattered spirit.
They prick my fingers.
The blood creates scars that grow numb.
That protect them,
but keep them from feeling.
As grief penetrates my soul,
deeper and deeper,
the scars grow thicker.
I cannot feel my heart beating.
I cannot hear my thoughts.
I cannot sense hunger or thirst.
Am I living or dead?
I cannot tell the difference.
There is no difference.

8

I did not sleep. I did not cry. I did not speak. A nurse came in and announced that I needed to eat something. Eat? How could she demand such a thing? The mere request sounded ridiculous. I mumbled a response and turned away from her. Eating is for the living. I was dead. I could see, but I couldn't hear or feel anything. Then, from the depths of my heart, I heard her voice whispering Peyton's name. As her soul left this world, Abby touched my heart with her tiny fingers and quietly reminded me that I could not be dead. Her sister needed me.

The nurse returned again, "Do you want to see her?"

A ridiculous question.

Within moments, she was there. The nurse walked into the room carrying a tiny blanket. As she came to the bedside, for just a brief second, my heart did not ache. Abby was swaddled just like every newborn, wearing a pink cap just like every newborn little girl. I held out my arms to take her and pull her to me. She was so tiny and so perfect. Her face was beautiful. She had a little button nose like Peyton's, and round little cheeks. I leaned down and softly kissed her perfect lips. I lingered there, hoping that by breathing gently into them, she would take in my breath, my life, and open her eyes.

I pulled my knees to my chest and gently laid her down on my legs. I unwrapped the blanket to see her. I wanted to take in every inch of her and burn it into my memory. Her little arms were muscular and her fingers were long, as were her legs. Each tiny finger and toe had a little nail. I looked for imperfections, but there were none. She was perfect and beautiful. I wrapped her in the blanket and held her to me. Jamie was content to sit with us, too broken to hold her. We marveled at her, telling one another how beautiful she was, how she looked like Peyton. I don't know how long we sat there, the three of us.

When it was finally time for her to go, I placed my lips to her ear and whispered, "Mommy and Daddy love you so much. We always will. And we will never forget you. That is my promise to you. You will be with us always in our hearts, and we will share you with those who loved you. We will make sure that

Peyton does not forget. My little angel, I am so sorry. I don't know why you must go. I love you."

And then she was gone.

Where are You, God?
As my heart wails in sorrow,
Sorrow and pain inflicted by You,
I cry out for comfort.
But You do not hear.
Or You do not listen.
Why have You abandoned me?
My soul knows the void left in Your wake.
Why did You forsake me?
Mortally wound me, then leave my soul to die.
I believed in You.
I trusted You.
I loved You.
I praised You.
Where are You?

9

January 10, 2003
2:00 PM

After staring out the window for hours, trying unsuccessfully to sleep, my little Princess walked through the door. "Hi, Mommy, are you okay?"

I breathed again.

As I held out my arms to embrace her, my voice broke with pain and joy, "Hi, Baby. I am so happy to see you. I've missed you. I'm okay, I just had a tummy ache, but I'll be able to come home soon. Climb up here and sit with me. I need a hug from my favorite girl."

She climbed onto the bed and curled up next to me. As I wrapped my arms around her, the pain in my heart eased. I could have sat like that forever.

We decided to wait and tell her what had happened when I could do it without completely breaking down. I did not want to be upset as I told her because I never wanted her to think that it was a sad thing to talk about Abby. I feared that if she thought it would make me sad, she would not talk about her and would want to forget. I also had not figured out how to explain this horror in a way that a three-year-old could understand. So for now, Mommy was simply sick and needed to be in the hospital for a little while.

She noticed the I.V. taped to my hand. "Did you have to get a shot?" she asked, her voice filled with concern.

I slid my hand under her, "Yes, baby, but it only hurt for a second. Tell me how school was today. What did you do?"

I did not look at Sue and Ted. I had seen the pain in their eyes and knew that I hung precariously to the façade of normalcy. One glance into their eyes would send me reeling over the edge. I could not do that in front of Peyton. So instead we made small talk. They each left the room several times, also barely hanging on. The inescapable heaviness overwhelmed them.

I know now that I should have asked Jamie to take Peyton to find a snack machine or a gift shop, to leave us for a while. But in the moment, she was my strength. As long as she was with me, I was alive. I needed her sweet smile and to hear her voice. The numbness created by the mix of indescribable grief and

Demerol closed my mind to any thoughts of others. I could only focus on trying to make it to the next moment, the next breath. Peyton was the source of my strength to do so. I realize now that I should have given Sue and Ted the chance to see Abby and say good-bye. But they did not ask, and I simply did not think of it.

Finally, they had to go. I wanted Peyton to stay with me, knowing that her absence would only create a bigger void in my heart, but she needed to go. The grief felt by the four of us was shrinking the room, stealing the air, and the façade was quickly vaporizing. After several kisses and promises that I would be home soon, my sweet girl left. As the door closed, my heart did not mercifully close with it. For a brief moment, the pain was so intense I believed that one could truly die of a broken heart.

January 10, 2003
5:00 PM

A few hours later, an official-looking woman walked through the door, "Mr. and Mrs. Stember? I am so sorry to bother you, but there is some information I need to give you. I know this is a very difficult time for you, but we need you to decide what you would like to do. You have the choice of either a burial or cremation. Because the hospital does not take care of the arrangements, you will have to do that yourselves. I have the names and phone numbers of several funeral homes in the area. Most all of them waive their fees for stillborns."

Stillborn. The word rolled around in my brain. That was something that happened to other people. My friend, Melissa's, sister-in-law had given birth just last year to stillborn twins. I remembered gasping in horror when she told me. "How awful. How can anyone endure such a thing?" I remembered thinking. That didn't happen to me.

The woman continued, "You just need to decide what you would like to do and then contact one of them. Unfortunately, you will need to let us know something by the time you leave the hospital tomorrow. If there is anything I can do to help, just let me know. I am also giving you the numbers of various agencies that can assist you with your grief. Is there a minister or rabbi that I can call for you?"

I regularly attended a church that I loved in Boynton Beach. Raised in a Southern Baptist church in Alabama, I first attended this Methodist Church because it was near my home. The first Sunday I visited, I immediately fell in love with its spirit. The sanctuary had yet to be built and we met in what was to become the classroom area once the money had been raised to complete the church. That first Sunday, I knew I had found my place.

Pastor Harold was a 39-year-old spit fire with five kids and boundless energy. A live wire, his sermons always spoke to me. But I did not want him called. I did not want to hear him tell me about God's will and how God would help us through this crisis. Pastor Harold was such a strong, wonderful Christian man. When he was in the room, you could feel God's presence and love. I was angry with God. He had taken my baby and abandoned me. I didn't want Him riding in with Pastor Harold and attempting to comfort me now. He had done this to us. He was all powerful. I had prayed, begged, pleaded. He could've given me back my Abby. He did not have to let her die.

"No," I replied.

"We have a minister here if you would like to have the baby baptized."

I did not see the point. Abby was dead. God had already taken her. But, for a reason that I could not discern, I wanted her to be baptized and treated with respect and dignity. I also wanted to see her again, "Okay."

The official-looking woman left. Within moments, another woman dressed in regular street clothes walked into the room, holding Abby. She smiled tenderly, "I'm the minister you asked for. Is this a good time?"

As if I could possibly turn her away as she stood there holding my daughter, I nodded. She slowly walked to the bed and sat down on the edge beside me. She cuddled Abby and gazed down at her, smiling. A sting pricked my heart.

"Can I hold her?" I asked. I wanted to look at her precious face again.

She gently handed her to me, careful to hold her head as though she were alive, "Yes. You can hold her as long as you would like. What is her name?"

"Abby."

"Abby," She repeated. "What a beautiful name for a beautiful girl." Then, she began talking to Abby, "Oh, Abby, beautiful, Abby. You are such a beautiful little angel."

This upset me immensely. It seemed patronizing and insincere. Suddenly, her presence was not welcomed. I pulled Abby to me protectively against this strange woman.

I had not noticed that she was also carrying a little vial of water. Holy or blessed water I assumed. She placed some on her finger and touched Abby's forehead. She formed the sign of the cross and said a prayer. I appreciated how gently she treated her, even though the whole thing seemed pointless. When she finished the ritual, she quietly stepped back and waited patiently for us to, once again, say good-bye. My heart was numb and my mind vacant. There was no pain or grief or tears, only disbelief. I offered Abby to her, and she received her softly. Cradling her, the minister seemed to rock Abby as she stepped away. As I watched them leave, I felt nothing.

Only a few friends visited: Montse, Michael, and Shawn.

Montse arrived first, sometime in the afternoon. A generation older than me, she was a wonderful friend and mother figure to me. Her husband, Hal, enjoyed the same relationship with Jamie. Despite our age differences, we had so many things in common. Jamie and Hal loved their planes and travel. Montse and I cherished our family and friends and devoured books. We spent many evenings at their home, eating and talking for hours. Montse showed such tenderness towards Peyton and always welcomed her with kisses, a special treat, and a movie.

Montse loved to entertain and always prepared a first-class spread, even if it was only for the five of us. Sophisticated and charming, she carried herself with such grace. Throughout their marriage, she and Hal had traveled the world many times over and were two of the most cultured people I had ever known. I loved them both, our relationship with them existing on two levels. We were close friends, but they were also parental in their affection, displaying the unconditional love and loyalty of family.

That afternoon, Montse and I spoke of everything; we spoke of nothing. She sat next to my bed and held my hand, gently stroking my fingers. A mother, she understood the unspeakable horror that we had just endured. We did not need to discuss it. Her presence, this time more maternal than friend, soothed me. She filled the void left in the wake of my mother's disease. The disease that robbed me of her and hid her from me, refusing to free her even for this moment, to sit next to my bed and hold my hand.

Michael arrived next. We had been friends for over ten years, having met in law school at Emory. He was one of my favorite people, freakishly intelligent and wickedly witty. We did not speak often, but when we did, the depth of our friendship prevented any awkwardness. Some people you just connect with, without the necessity of time to form a friendship. We had that, solidified by ten years.

During college, he slowly lost his father to cancer. The suffering and death of his Dad created both a deep-rooted anger and a child-like vulnerability. Michael assumed the pain of those he loved and bore it as an albatross. Not knowing what to say as he now sat by my bed, we spoke of family and other things, even laughing at times. His visit was a pleasant distraction, which Jamie also appreciated.

Finally, Shawn stopped by. Jamie and Shawn had been friends since high school, then attended college together. They joined the same fraternity and studied the same major, which threw them together often. Their experiences formed an indelible bond. Fiercely loyal, Shawn, too, shared his friends' joys and sorrows as if they were his own. When he marched into the room, tears filled his eyes. He grabbed Jamie, hugged him hard, and immediately began cursing. He was genuinely angry and sad. It touched me and made me love him even more.

No one else came. I could not understand why. I knew that our friends and family loved us and were not intentionally hurting us, but their absence was painful. I felt abandoned. The silence in the room as Jamie and I sat alone, too pained to speak, only added to the heaviness in our hearts. Why did no one come? Did they think we needed time? Privacy? Space? Or did they simply not know what to say or do? Was it all too uncomfortable? I didn't begrudge anyone or impute bad intentions, but the loneliness was almost unbearable.

I needed to go home, to be with Jamie and Peyton.

There is no dignity in death.

10

After a restless night, despite the Ambien, we again sat alone. The hours crept by as we waited for the doctor to discharge me. We turned on the television to fill the silence because we could not speak. Yet still, no one came. I stared at the ceiling, counting the specks in the panels.

Shortly before noon, Dr. Kaufman, the on-call doctor, arrived. After several questions and a quick exam, he agreed to let me go home. I felt such relief. I needed to get away from that room. We were captives in the place where the most horrific thing that had ever happened to us had occurred. They had not even asked if we wanted to change rooms after Abby's birth. They simply left us there, in that tomb.

As we packed, the official-looking woman knocked on the door, "Mr. and Mrs. Stember? I'm sorry to bother you again. I was told that you are being discharged. We still don't know what you intend to do as far as your baby's arrangements. Have you made a decision? Did you have an opportunity to call any of the funeral homes?"

"No," Jamie answered. "Would you please give us a few minutes?"

"Yes, of course. I'll come back and check on you in a little while."

After she left, Jamie turned to me, "Do you know what you want to do?"

My mind was spinning. I truly did not know what I wanted to do. I didn't want to do anything. Should we have a burial or a cremation? I could not endure either choice. Each slashed open my heart.

In my mind, I saw the tiny coffins we would be shown, their size alone creating indescribable agony. Then there would be a service, with soft music and prayer and a minister speaking of God's will and how He would comfort us in our time of grief. The very thought made me angry. Then we would be forced to watch as the tiny casket was carried to her graveside. Our little angel would be either placed in the ground with dirt dumped on top of her, or walled up in a mausoleum. Burial was an option only if I could be with her. Cradling her in my arms. I could not allow her to be alone under the Earth.

The other option was more gut-wrenching. Her little body set on a pyre and burned slowly to a painfully small pile of ash. Her bones crumbled and mutilated. My fingers began to tingle and I couldn't see. White spots appeared in front of my eyes. My stomach churned. I could not think. I could not hear.

Jamie pleaded. "Lesa? Are you okay? What do you think, honey?"

I just stared at him. "Honey, I can't…"

"What do you want to do?" he pleaded, needing me to help him with this tremendous decision and tell him what I wanted. He couldn't do this alone. I couldn't force him to do this alone. To bear the weight of this decision. But I wanted neither choice. I couldn't help him. I couldn't tell him what to do. I looked at him, tears streaming down my face.

My heart thumped in my ears, "Honey, I can't. I don't know. I'm sorry. What do you want to do?"

He knew. He did not hesitate, "I want to have her cremated. I can't handle a burial and service. I was thinking that we could take her to California."

I knew exactly what he was saying to me. We had gone to Northern California on our honeymoon and stayed several days in San Francisco and Monterey. We spent an entire afternoon driving through Pebble Beach, stopping and marveling at each of the tourist stops along the Seventeen-Mile Drive. We had agreed that it was the most beautiful place on Earth and that one day we would have a home there. A glimpse of Heaven, its beauty is unparalleled.

I met his gaze and our hearts were one, "Okay."

And it was done. He picked up the phone and called the first name on the list, which was a funeral home just down the road in Boca. As I listened to him, my love for him grew. At that moment, I could not speak. It was tormenting to even hear the conversation. Yet, he was handling things and making the arrangements all by himself. I had no strength to give him. Instead, I kept taking his, which was unfair. He needed me just as much as I needed him, but I had nothing to give. I only took.

Just before we left, the nurse came in with the discharge papers. As she droned on, I heard none of the instructions she read to me. She paused as if to steel herself and continued, "I have a few things to give you. First, I have a folder for you with information about grief support groups. There are many resources out there that can be helpful. You should contact one of them when you are ready. I also have a couple of pictures that we took of your daughter, as well as her footprints."

"Thank you."

I took the pictures and studied them. They did not look like Abby. The baby in the pictures looked like a doll with a red, distorted face. I had memorized every inch of Abby's face as I held her. The pictures looked nothing like her. I wished we had taken our own pictures. At the time it had seemed inappropriate some-how, but now, it was yet another regret.

When I looked at the footprints, my heart broke again. They were so tiny, but so powerful. To me, they were evidence that she had been with us. Those tiny footprints from the tiny feet that had touched our hearts, leaving their imprint forever. I traced each toe with my fingertip and remembered how often I had felt these tiny feet kick me. These tiny feet that let me know she was alive. I so wanted to hear the footfall of these tiny feet. How could I not have known when they grew still that something terrible had happened to her?

The nurse then grabbed a wheelchair I had not noticed, "I have to wheel you out, I'm sorry. Hospital policy."

I obediently sat down in the chair. As she wheeled me through the maternity ward, I heard newborn cries and happy voices. I saw a new father carrying flow-ers. The joy of these new families only intensified my heartache. My arms throbbed with emptiness.

The nurse deposited me on the front walkway where I waited while Jamie went to retrieve the car. I had dreamed of this day since learning I was pregnant. The day I would leave West Boca having given birth to Abby. The reality was nothing like the dream. I sat there, alone, waiting for Jamie with my empty hands folded in my lap, wishing, once again, that I could disappear.

As we drove down Glades Room toward home, I noticed through the car win-dow that the world simply went about its day. There was a line in the McDonald's drive-through. A state trooper had pulled over a speeding car. Peo-ple were pulling into the Publix parking lot to do their grocery shopping. I grew angry. I wanted to roll down the window and scream, "How can you just go about your day as if nothing has happened? My baby is dead. Don't any of you care that my baby is dead?" The daily routines of these strangers offended me. My anger towards God grew. I prayed, "So this is how it is? A baby dies and no one notices. The world just keeps on turning. You are so cruel."

Friends choose to love you.
Choose to give you their strength when you have none.
Choose to hold you and absorb your pain,
as your tears saturate their hearts.
Friends choose to bear their souls
and allow you to see their suffering,
so you do not feel alone in your own.
Friends choose to climb into that dark place of your sorrow.
To lay with you in its depths,
hold your hand,
and gently guide you back to life.
Friends choose to love you.

11

"Mommy!"

Against doctor's orders not to lift anything, I scooped my sweet angel into my arms. She wrapped her little arms around me and squeezed. Paisley and Taylor jumped up at me, squealing in delight. It felt good to be home.

"How's your tummy, Mommy?"

I kissed her little cheeks, "Much better, baby. How are you? I missed you so much!"

"I missed you, too, Mommy." Then her little hand caressed my belly, "Hi, Baby Abby."

My knees weakened and my chest tightened. I fought the tears defiantly slipping from my eyes. I carried her to the couch, where we sat cuddling and reading until she grew bored and ran off to her room to play. I closed my eyes and sighed, allowing my mind to go blank.

Then, the doorbell rang. The dogs predictably went bananas, barking and spinning in circles. Paisley ran and slammed himself into the front door. When I opened it, a tremendous bouquet blinded me. I peered around it and saw Leslie. She stormed into the house, followed by Terri, Lauren, and Donnie carrying little Nicholas. Grocery bags spilled out of Leslie and Terri's arms. Leslie kissed me, "Sweetie, I hope you don't mind us coming. We wanted to see you." Did I mind?

Terri hugged me tightly, balancing the groceries, "I hope it's okay that I brought Nick." Nicholas was only eights months old. She later confessed her apprehension in bringing him, fearing that seeing a baby would upset me. Seeing Nick could never upset me. He was a beautiful, sweet little boy. I assured her that I appreciated Nicky's presence, and her concern. He made me smile, as did Ms. Lauren. Peyton and Lauren were five months apart and met when Peyton was only six weeks old. They were the best of friends. When Peyton saw Lauren, she screamed in delight and grabbed her hand, then pulled her into her room to play. Hearing their giggles brought comfort.

I followed Leslie and Terri into the kitchen where they dropped the groceries onto the counter. The bags overflowed with homemade frozen dinners and other treats. Leslie opened the freezer and moved things around, "We didn't want you to have to worry about dinner for a while. I made some homemade lasagna and a casserole. Terri picked out some goodies for Peyton. The stuff Lauren likes. We'll find room for it in here."

Flowers and food were the traditional offerings of friends comforting mourners. This acknowledgement by my friends, this recognition of Abby's life and death, touched me deeply. I whispered, "Thank you."

We moved to the living room where we watched the kids play. No one asked what had happened over the last two days. No one needed details. They openly surrounded us with their love, which eased the grief smothering our hearts. We chatted about nothing until Tye and Kelly arrived. Kelly's face wore a tense expression and her eyes were bloodshot. Speechless, she looked to Leslie and Terri. I stood and embraced her.

"It's going to be okay," I reassured her as she quietly cried. My friends truly mourned and their sorrow moved me.

She stepped back and looked into my eyes, "What happened?"

I could not meet her gaze and glanced away, "They don't know, Kel. Nothing was wrong with her. The cord wasn't around her neck. I hadn't been sick. They just don't know. They drew blood, mine and hers, so maybe the answer's there. I don't know..."my voice faded.

Terri placed her hand on me as Leslie asserted, "They'll find out. Don't you worry. There must be a reason."

I attempted a smile. "No they won't," my mind screamed. "There is no answer. There is no reason. It just is."

Leslie, Terri, Kelly and I moved to the bedroom and climbed onto my bed, leaving the boys in the living room with the kids. We sat in a circle and talked about nothing. Sitting there, I felt strong, like I could survive. Their love and friendship gave me strength and a sense of hope crept into my heart. When they finally left hours later, a vacuum sucked that strength out behind them.

I suddenly realized how very tired I was, having forgotten the physical toll my body had endured. Thankfully, it was time for Peyton's afternoon nap. I welcomed not only resting but also holding Peyton and stroking her hair in the solitude of my room as she drifted off to sleep. I slid under the covers with her and draped my arm over her. Fatigue weighed down my body and my mind grew numb, but I was unable to sleep. I listened to her rhythmic breathing, trying to lose myself in it. When I was certain she was sleeping, I silently cried.

I lay there until I heard voices. Sliding out of bed, I tucked the covers back under Peyton and went into our bathroom to splash water on my burning eyes. I was frightened by what I saw. I did my best to erase the signs of fatigue and sobbing, brushed my hair, and quietly snuck out of the room and back into the living room. Michael was there with his wife, Melissa, and their son, Jackson, sitting on the patio with Jamie and his parents. As I slid open the patio door, Melissa stood and embraced me. She touched my face, "Hi, baby, how are you?"

"Okay," I lied. "Thank you guys for coming."

Michael squeezed me, "Of course we came."

Again, no one asked what had happened. They just wanted to love us, give us strength, and offer their prayers and help.

That afternoon, the flowers and cards began arriving, containing kind words of comfort and condolence. The cards were difficult to read, but I cherished knowing that our family and friends thought of us. Their absence at the hospital had not been born of indifference but of respect and a misguided belief that we needed solitude. Each sympathy card reaffirmed Abby's life and acknowledged the fact that her death was the death of a child to be grieved and missed.

A small package arrived from Scott and Erin, our friends who lived just outside of Atlanta. Jamie met Scott at Florida State when Jamie joined Scott's fraternity. Their solid friendship survived the after-life of college. I had met Scott and Erin at their wedding in 1997. During the reception, Jamie caught Erin's garter and I caught her bouquet. Two years later at our wedding, they teased that they were the reason we ended up together.

Just three months earlier, we had visited them at their home when I was eleven weeks pregnant with Abby. They shared our excitement about our growing family. They loved parenthood and their two children were the center of their world. Erin, who had taken time off from her successful marketing career to stay home with them, was an amazing woman, creative and full of energy. As was Scott. They seized life and were so easy to be with. "Good people" we called them.

As I now opened their condolence package, I pulled out a card and two small candles. Perplexed, I opened the card.

Jamie, Lesa & Peyton,

After trying to find a card with the "right" words, we clearly understood that there is nothing we can really say to help you, but we do want to let you know that we are thinking about all of you and keeping you in our prayers. We are sending lots of love, compassion, & strength and we hope you can feel it through the pain. We have enclosed two candles—one we thought you could light on what should have been her birthday. Although we were not lucky enough to meet her, she certainly was alive within the two of you and will live on in your hearts and in Heaven.

The second candle is for Peyton—that she may continue to be a light for you to get through this. We are so blessed with what God does give us but it never seems fair what He takes home to Him. She will be an angel now for all of you.

We love you and will keep you in our prayers,

Scott, Erin, Jameson & J.D.

A short time later, my parents arrived. They had driven most of the night from Alabama, stopping only for a few hours of sleep. I struggled to swallow my tears as Dad hugged me tightly. Funny how even as an adult, my Dad could invoke child-like feelings in me. I then looked into Mom's eyes. I knew she did not fully comprehend what had happened, but I could see sadness. Despite the fact that her disease had taken her from me, something deep inside of her connected to my pain. When she said, "Hi baby" she was there for a fleeting second. My Mom. I wanted to fall into her arms like a child.

After small talk about their drive and their night, I confided in my Dad, sharing with him some of the excruciating details no one else had heard. He listened patiently, the words obviously hurting him not only because he had lost a grandchild, but because of my pain.

I held my breath, then whispered, "They took pictures of her." The words stung.

His eyes widened in disbelief, "They did?" At first thought, the idea seemed irreverent and unnatural.

I put my hand on his arm, reassuring him, "They don't look like her, though. I don't understand that. How could they be pictures of her? Would you like to see them?"

"Yes," he released the breath he had been holding. His instinctive horror was shadowed by my need to share the pictures with him, and his need to see them.

"Okay. They're in the bedroom."

I tiptoed into our bedroom so as not to disturb my sleeping princess and pulled the folder the hospital had given us off the dresser. I opened it to grab the pictures and the tiny footprints confronted me. I eased them from the folder, along with the pictures, then quietly slid back out of the room.

Dad's voice quivered as he clenched the tiny footprints, "They're so small."

"I know, Daddy. Aren't they perfect?"

"They are." His voice betrayed his struggle as he tried to reconcile their apparent representation of her life with knowing that they were placed there in her death. We sat still and reverent for several moments. Finally, he asked, "Can I see the pictures?"

I handed them to him, "She was so much more beautiful than in these pictures. I don't understand that."

He quietly stared until the silence was broken by the bedroom door opening. My sleepy girl emerged, rubbing her eyes, "Granddaddy? Nana?" She climbed into my lap, confused. I slid the pictures and the footprints under a magazine, not wanting Peyton to see them. I pulled her to me tightly and rocked her. We all peacefully watched as the sun faded.

That night after Peyton had fallen asleep and Jamie was showering, I stretched across the bed. My maternity pants slid down and I jerked them up in anger. I was forced to wear them as my belly shrunk, but they were ill-fitting and taunted me. I sighed and rolled over onto my back where my eyes were drawn to the bedside table. I noticed the journal that Melissa had given me for my birthday four months earlier. We had been friends for many years and she knew I loved writing. She also knew I had neglected my passion in the wake of marriage and motherhood. Her gift was meant to encourage me, but its pages remained clean. I grabbed it and began writing without thinking. The words pouring from my pen flowed not from my mind but from my broken soul. The crushing weight of my pain grew lighter as I wrote:

January 11, 2003

My Dearest Abby,

I so looked forward to giving birth to you. I daydreamed about it from the day I found out you were with me. I imagined you being placed in my arms, eyes squinting from your first glimpses of light. Hearing you cry. I so longed to hear you cry. But your birth was not as I had dreamed. You were swaddled and placed in my arms, but there were no cries from your little lungs, and no tears of joy. Only silence and the most unimaginable sadness. I had never seen your Daddy cry until the day you came into this world. I held you-so tiny and so still. I wanted to look into your eyes, but they were closed forever.

Only a few days before, I felt you inside me, moving and kicking. You were so alive. Why did you have to go? Why didn't I get to see your smile? Or your eyes? I'm sure they are beautiful pools of blue like your big sister's. She wanted to meet you so badly. She talks about you all the time. She wanted bunk beds so she could sleep above you. She felt you, too. Just the other day she asked me to wake you so she could feel you move in my belly. She loves you even though she hasn't met you. She told me that she was going to let you have her Little Pooh, her most prized and loved toy. I don't know how I will ever explain to her that she won't meet you. She already loved you.

I am so sorry that my body betrayed you. You were so perfect. For some reason, my body could not hold you. I am so sorry, my beautiful angel. My arms ache with emptiness. Words cannot describe how my heart breaks. I love you so much. Please forgive me for not being able to bring you into this world to meet your big sister. And the Mommy and Daddy who wanted you so much. I will never forget your angelic face and how perfect you are. You will be with me always.

I love you,
Mommy.

A solitary seed of anger in my heart.
It was not planted,
or purposefully placed there.
It fell.
Scattered from the explosion in my soul.
The shattering of my spirit.
Firmly rooted,
it grows.
Showered by my unending tears,
until it fully blooms.
It creeps into the crevices of my heart,
consuming it.
It crawls up my throat.
I can taste its bitterness on my tongue.
It flushes over my face,
into my eyes,
blinding me with rage.
My spirit will not know peace
until it is purged from my soul.

12

The next morning after breakfast, Jamie dressed to go to the funeral home to finalize Abby's arrangements. He announced, "There's no need for you to go. I can handle this by myself. You just stay here with your folks and Peyton."

I knew he was trying to protect me, but I could not allow him to go alone. Abby was his baby, too. He was suffering just as much as me and, despite his assertion, I knew he needed me with him.

"No, I'm going with you," I asserted.

He protested, "Honey, you really don't need to. I will take care of it."

"I know you will, but I want to go." I didn't want to imply that he didn't have the strength to protect me so I confided that I wanted to see her again, "Maybe they'll let us see her. I need to see her again. I was so drugged out before."

He pulled me to him, "Okay. If you think you really want to. Will Peyton be alright with your Dad?"

"Yeah, he'll keep her busy."

I went to the kitchen and found Dad pouring another cup of coffee. "Daddy, Jamie and I have to go to the funeral home. Will you be okay here with Mom and Peyton?"

"Sure, baby. But why don't you let me go with Jamie? He can't go by himself, but you shouldn't go." He, too, needed to protect me. I was still his little girl. I also knew that he hoped to see her. By holding him back and not allowing him to come right away, I had deprived him of seeing her in the hospital.

"No, Daddy. I need to go. She was my baby," my voice cracked. I stared at the ceiling, willing the tears away. "I know you want to see her. If they let us, I'll tell them that you're going to come later today to see her, okay?"

"Okay, baby. I understand."

We kissed Peyton good-bye then drove away in silence, not knowing what to say. The funeral home was only ten minutes away, but the drive seemed shorter. There was not enough time to prepare ourselves for what we were about to do. The parking lot was empty and I wondered if anyone was there. Jamie assured me that he had spoken with one of the owners and even though it was Sunday, some-one would meet us. He pulled into a space and took the keys from the ignition. I closed my eyes and took a deep breath, bracing myself. After climbing out, I grabbed Jamie's hand for strength and he looked at me tenderly. The bond between us solidified more with each step we took towards that awful place.

A kind face greeted us and ushered us into an office. As Jamie spoke with the owner, my eyes surveyed the room. There were plaques with accolades of kindness and professional service, a few paintings, and boxes of tissues stashed in strategic places. Then, my stomach lurched. There were urns subtly displayed as merchandise, unobtrusively sitting on a shelf. I covered my mouth in an attempt to squelch the sickness creeping up my throat.

"No," Jamie was saying, "We don't need anything else. We plan on scattering her ashes so we don't need an urn. Whatever you give us will be sufficient." His voice was strong, with no hint of the searing pain he was certainly feeling. He turned to me, "Honey, do you have any questions?"

I had heard nothing of their conversation. I searched the floor, gathering my strength, and then whimpered, "Can I see her?"

The owner softly answered, "I'm sorry, but no. Her body isn't here. She's at our facility in Lake Worth."

I could not conceal my shock, "She isn't here? But I wanted to see her!"

"I'm so sorry." Then, to my disbelief, he unnecessarily continued, "Even if she were here, we wouldn't recommend a viewing. She will not look the way you remember her because she has been with us for a few days."

"What do you mean?" The fact that these details were merciless and unnecessary escaped me. "Why would she look different?"

I had been to many open casket funerals. The dead always looked different, but not unrecognizable.

Bluntly, he explained, "Because her body has been kept at a cold temperature."

The disgust struck me and my head spun. She was going to be cremated. There was no need to embalm her. She was lying in a refrigerator, waiting to be placed on a pyre and dissolved to ash. The indignity of it sickened me. The image brutally clawed its way to the front of my mind despite my efforts to push it away. Emotion overwhelmed me. My soul screamed at God, "Why do we have to endure this? Why are You doing this to us? This is so horrible. So wretched. It was hard enough to lose her, but to subject her to this indignity. Why?"

I searched my mind frantically for a better way. There must be some other way. Sadly, I realized that there is no dignity in death. Defeated, I rose to my feet and walked out the door, saying nothing. As we drove home, I rested my head on my knees.

Jamie touched my back. "Are you okay?"

I didn't look up. "No. You?"

"No."

Dad and I spent the rest of the day watching Peyton and Mom play. Not as a grandmother and her grandchild, but as two children. Mom's decline was ever more apparent. My inability to collapse into her arms was yet another loss to endure. My mind mercifully shut down again and a numbness enveloped me. I had no desire to eat, no desire to sleep, and no desire to speak. But I could not leave Peyton. She needed me. Watching my Mom, it became poignantly obvious just how much a daughter needs her mother. For Peyton, for Jamie, for my Dad, I would not leave.

Tuesday morning after starting the coffee, I decided to shower while Peyton lay in bed with Jamie and watched Disney Channel. She loved climbing into bed with us in the early morning and snuggling under the covers, drinking apple juice and watching "The Book of Pooh." As I undressed, my chest ached, as it had since I was released from the hospital. I assumed I had injured it thrashing around during labor. It had been a strange soreness, almost muscular, that made breathing a little painful. This morning's soreness was different, more of a throbbing, but I thought nothing of it.

I stepped into the shower and slipped under the water, welcoming its warmth as it melted some of my fatigue. Suddenly, my breasts started to tingle. I glanced down, stifling a scream. Milk. No one had warned me, although I should have known. I'd given birth before. Giving birth to Abby had flipped a hormonal switch that caused my oblivious body to prepare to feed her. I slid to the floor of the shower, my tears mingling with the warm water. In the seclusion of the shower, I surrendered to my despair. My sobs muffled.

From Heaven,
You peered down and chose me.
Trusted me with your life.
To be your vessel to this Earth.
You stirred inside of me.
Nestled into my body.
Into my heart.
But my body betrayed you.
And me.
Rejecting you.
Killing you.
My guilt consumes me.
Crushing me.
Blinding me.
Killing me.
As it should.

13

Friday marked one week since Abby's birth and death. It was also our fourth wedding anniversary. Everyone encouraged us to go out to dinner, but it seemed disrespectful and inappropriate. How could we go to dinner and celebrate so soon? I had no desire to go. Food repulsed me and I couldn't amass the energy required for small talk. But I knew Jamie needed and wanted to go. He had asked several times and I had responded with ambivalence. He needed something positive to grasp, and needed a break from the sorrow that penetrated every pore of our home and our lives. So I agreed.

That afternoon, I decided to explain to Peyton what had happened. She was not quite three, but she was sensitive and keenly attuned to my moods. She heard the whispers and watched us plod around the house, lifeless and robotic. I wanted to explain to her why we were sad and make certain that she knew it was nothing she had done. Children live in a very small world in which they are the center, creating a sense of responsibility for bad things that happen.

I pulled her into our bedroom, away from the distractions of her toys and the television. "Pey Pey, I need to talk to you about something important."

Her big blue eyes widened, "Okay, Mommy."

I hesitated, searching for the right words, "Do you remember when Mommy had to go to the hospital last week?"

"Yeah. Your tummy hurt."

I took her into my lap, "Yes, baby. Well, it was more than a tummy ache. I had Baby Abby."

"You had Baby Abby? Where is she? When is she coming home?"

I began stroking her hair, pushing it behind her ears and out of her eyes. "She's not, baby."

"Why not?" Her little brow furrowed and I saw confusion in her eyes. "Why isn't she coming home?"

My stomach tightened and I forced myself to breathe. "Well, baby, she was very sick and she died. Do you know what that means?"

"No, Mommy. What is that?"

How to explain this escaped me, but I tried, "It means that she was too sick to come home. Instead she went to live in Heaven."

Anger replaced her confusion, "Heaven? Why did she have to go live in Heaven? She's supposed to live here. Where is Heaven?"

I fought to maintain my even tone, "Up in the sky where God lives. She's an angel now, like a bird. You can talk to her whenever you want. You may not see her, but she will hear you."

I led her to the window and lifted her up. "Talk to her just like you did when she was in my belly. Just look up in the sky, into the clouds, and talk to her."

She cocked her little head and squinted her eyes, searching, "Oh. Look, Mommy, in the clouds. Hi, Baby Abby."

"Yes, baby. Just like that." I held her tightly, hiding my face so that she would not see my tears. I never wanted her to think that speaking of Abby made me sad for fear that she would stop. I knew that she didn't understand. Death is too abstract for a three-year-old. It's too abstract for anyone, actually. But she understood that Abby was no longer in my belly and would not be coming home.

Later that afternoon, Jamie and I decided to invite Bob and Pat to our anniversary outing, which would force us to speak. Had we gone alone, we would have peered over our food and failed miserably at pretending to enjoy the evening. With Bob and Pat, we could focus on others for a while. Sue and Ted offered to baby-sit, to spend time with Peyton. They needed to include themselves in our lives, to ease their own pain with Peyton's smile. They, too, were hurting. Our exclusion of them had not been designed to further hurt them, but their pain was discernable and added to the grief that permeated our home. They wanted only to help us and be allowed to grieve with us, but it was simply too difficult.

When they arrived, their faces wore genuine smiles. They were thrilled to see Peyton and to be invited back into our lives. I, too, was happy they were there. I loved them deeply and missed them. They settled onto the couch, reassuring us that we should take as long as we liked and try to enjoy the night. This seemed an impossible undertaking to me, but I smiled in agreement.

Peyton followed me into the bedroom to watch me dress. She was happy that Grandma and Poppy were there to play with her, but also apprehensive about my leaving. We had not been apart since I had come home from the hospital. An inexplicable sense of doom blanketed my heart, creating a fear that Peyton would be taken from me, too, if she were out of my sight. My paranoia caused me to keep her home from preschool the entire week. The thought of dropping her off and leaving her for even a few hours created an intense anxiety. I didn't think,

"She could be hurt and need me." My thoughts were morbid. I feared that if she left my sight, I would never see her again.

As Peyton and I stood in my closet, I dismissed my fear. Jamie needed to do this. He needed to celebrate our anniversary and escape reality for a few hours. So against every maternal instinct, I dressed. Instead of wearing maternity clothes, I decided to attempt my regular clothes. I assured myself that they could not possibly fit. Only seven days ago, I had been six months pregnant. I pulled a pair of pants from the back of my closet and tried them on. To my disbelief, they fit. How was that possible? How could my body go back to "normal" so quickly? I felt betrayed by it. Only a few days ago, it produced milk and now I was climbing back into my regular clothes. How could my body have forgotten her so quickly?

Two days later, I picked up my journal again.

January 19, 2003

Over the past nine days, I have felt closer to Jamie than I have in such a long time. We have a tendency to get caught up in the daily minutia and take one another for granted. But these past nine days, I have wanted nothing more than to hold his hand, to be close to him.

Peyton has been the glue that has kept my sanity together, but Jamie has been my strength. He has sacrificed leaning on me in order to be strong for me. I have seen such love and tenderness in his eyes. He's such a "man's man" and sometimes I feel that I miss out on his tenderness and affection. But since Abby died, I have felt so much love from him. So much tenderness and strength. It isn't in what he says or does. It is simply in the way he looks at me. He looks at me with these eyes that are full of love and concern. I feel safe.

I only regret that I am unable to reciprocate his strength. I fear that when he looks at me, he sees only eyes full of pain, fear, and desperation. I know that he is mourning, too, and I regret that I only take his strength and am not there for him. Every day I am reminded of his love and how blessed I am to have him for a husband.

My sweet PeyPey is so perfect. Before this tragedy, I loved her more than I thought was ever possible. I now love her so much that it physically hurts. I can't imagine focusing my life on anything else. I just hope that I am able to tame myself so that I don't crush her with the weight of my love for her.

And my dear Abby. She has changed my forever. When I lost my other two babies this year, I mourned them. I loved them and the idea of them. But having lost them at seven weeks, I did not know them. I knew my sweet Abby. I saw her take shape every week and heard her heartbeat. I felt those first butterfly flutters, then the kicks. Peyton and Jamie felt them, too. She was alive. My body changed, my belly protruding as she grew. She was so much a part of our family already. I thought of myself as a Mommy of children and we would refer to "the girls." I can't believe that she isn't going to be a part of our daily lives.

I will never get to rock her to sleep, to feed her a bottle. I had pictured her sweet face, holding her when she was born. Crying hysterically from the joy of her cry and knowing that she was finally safe. Instead, I cried hysterically because she was born asleep, with her eyes closed. I will never see those beautiful eyes or feel her tiny fingers wrap around mine. I will never hear her cry or call me "Mommy." I will never again kiss those perfect lips or feel her breath on my chest. I will never feel those tiny feet kick me again.

I am sure that she is in Heaven with her two brothers or sisters, looking down on us and wishing we were not so sad. I can't believe that I am the mother of four children and will only know one. I hope that my sweet Peyton can handle all the love that she will certainly know.

Purgatory.
The place that is neither Heaven, nor Hell, nor Earth.
Where one is neither dead nor alive,
But instead waits.
Why would God create such a place?
Why prolong the suffering of death?
The suspension of time and resolution.
The agony of death stretched thin,
the seconds slowed to an excruciating pace.
Waiting in that place between what life was and what it will be without you.

14

Jamie and I agreed that we would take Abby's ashes to California that week. The thought of bringing them home and having them around the house made me very uncomfortable. Where to put them? On a shelf? A bookcase? In the closet? Any location seemed trivial and unworthy. To release her right away felt right. The funeral home assured us that she would be ready in a matter of days.

We called Sue and Ted to ask if they could baby-sit our puppies for the few days we would be gone. We had not shared our plans with anyone and the news came as a shock to them. To us, deciding to have Abby cremated and then taking her to California seemed an intensely private decision. Our hearts were so broken that the idea of sharing these moments, these decisions, never formed in our minds. We felt the loss so deeply that we clung to one another. Sharing with others only intensified the pain.

Jamie's parents and my Dad all listened without comment to our decision. Appreciating our pain, they did not make their own needs known. They did not insist on a burial and a place to visit. They simply supported our decision and offered to do whatever we needed. Not including them would become yet another regret.

Ted and Sue agreed to keep our dogs. They also offered to have Peyton stay with them, insisting that she would be better staying in Florida, going to pre-school, and playing with her friends. No need to drag her across the country, to subject her to what we were doing. Jamie considered the idea, uncertain as to how we would include her without exposing her.

For me, there was no discussing it. I could not leave her behind. My impending sense of doom increased my paranoia about Peyton's safety. I could not leave her for four days. She certainly would not be there when I returned. Something terrible would happen and would take her from me. She had to stay with us. Jamie and I would make certain that she would not see Abby's ashes and would not understand what was happening. But when she was older and all grown up, we would share with her what had happened and maybe she would remember being there.

We planned to leave on January 22nd. We had both been given only two weeks leave from work and decided to spend the last days of that leave in California. We also wanted to be back before Peyton's third birthday. We checked the flights on American, planning to use our travel privileges, and made reservations at a hotel in Monterey. There would be two days of travel, and two days in California. We were not yet certain as to our plan, knowing only that Monterey was the most beautiful place on Earth and the closest thing to Heaven. We would know what to do when we got there. Abby would tell us.

Jamie called the funeral home. It had been ten days since Abby's death and we had not been called. They promised him we could pick her up the next day. My mind reeled as I pictured what was occurring. They still had not cremated her? She was still lying in a freezer, blue and preserved? The thought made my skin crawl. What were they waiting for? There is no dignity in death.

She was not ready the next day. We kept calling and finally told them that we were going to California, and why. They told us that we could pick up her the next morning, the morning we planned to fly out of Miami. It seemed excruciating and just another thing gone wrong. In retrospect, it probably saved my sanity to not have her ashes sitting on the bedroom dresser or shoved in the closet out of sight, waiting.

The next morning, we phoned the funeral home to make certain she was ready. After they assured us that she was, we quickly and quietly packed. The anticipation of what was about to occur settled into the pit of my stomach. Abby's death was not one moment in time, but a series of events that continued to flog us. Each day was a new horrible step in the process. My mind and heart grew more numb with each new wave of pain.

We climbed into Jamie's car, a two-door Honda Prelude, and strapped Peyton into her car seat in the miniature back seat. She giggled and playfully placed her hands on the window above her, excited that we were going on a trip. I settled into the passenger's seat and steeled myself. We had agreed that I would wait in the car with Peyton while Jamie went into the funeral home. There was no need to drag her inside and have to explain to her where we were and what we were doing. Waiting in the car allowed us to pretend as though it were just another day.

We pulled into the parking lot, which was full. This struck me as tragic. Either there was an abundance of death or a funeral. Jamie drove around to the rear and parked in an adjacent lot. Peyton, enthralled with her ability to touch the roof of the compact car, did not realize when Jamie snuck away. As soon as he disappeared from sight, I began watching for him in the side mirror. My stomach churned and my eyes stung. I fought the tears, refusing to give into the grief overwhelming me. I knew that if I released a single tear, they would not cease and Peyton would not understand why.

I stared at the mirror, tuning out Peyton's singing. The innocence and joy in her voice was a stark contrast to my dark soul. After what seemed an eternity, Jamie emerged from the side of the building carrying a small, brown, unobtrusive box. I looked away, choking on my tears. I could not contain them any longer. The trunk creaked open and, seconds later, slammed shut. He appeared at the driver's door, empty handed, then slid into the seat without a word and jerked the car into gear. I sobbed, unable to control myself. The thought of Abby in the trunk crushed me. What was left of her little body sitting in the trunk of our car. There is no dignity in death.

Fear creates chaos.
What was once ordered,
predictable,
normal,
now in great disarray.
I search my mind,
trying to control my thoughts,
my fear,
the consuming panic.
I cannot find my way through my violated mind.
I trip over my jumbled thoughts in the infinite space.
An abyss without form or boundaries.
Or end.

15

Jamie fumbled with the radio, searching through the incessant morning talk-show nonsense for music. I struggled to regain control, choking down my sobs. Peyton continued to sing and chat aimlessly as she placed her palms on the windows, smearing tiny handprints. Jamie and I stared ahead, incapable of small talk. The radio brought solace as music finally filled the car. My mind churned the image of Abby's ashes in the trunk, bouncing and sliding around.

When we arrived at Miami International Airport, Jamie dropped us at the terminal entrance. The stench of exhaust and cigarettes saturated the air. As Jamie hoisted our bags from the trunk, I averted my eyes, unaware that he had knowingly hid the brown box in his suitcase, snug and warm amidst his clothes. I grabbed Peyton's car seat, which I carefully balanced on top of my suitcase, and wheeled them inside, guiding Peyton through the crowd with my other hand. The volume of people frightened me as the kaleidoscope through which I now viewed the world twisted. These strangers were all latent kidnappers, child molesters, and psychotics who preyed on children. I clenched her hand and drew her close to my side. The chaos required focus and granted a reprieve from my thoughts.

Waiting for Jamie to return from parking the car, I protectively backed Peyton into the wall, shielding her with my body. My eyes surveyed everyone. Finally, he appeared and we fell in line at security. I hid the fear in my voice as I continuously called to Peyton to stand next to me. She insisted on dodging back and forth under the security rope, stopping to twirl on the posts until it was our turn to walk through the gates.

As we collected our things on the other side, one of the agents bellowed, "Sir, wait one moment. I need to talk to you. You have something suspicious in your bag."

Realizing immediately what was about to happen, Jamie turned to me with a pained expression, "Go. Go wait for me in the chairs in front of the escalator."

My mind did not register what was happening. "Okay," I obeyed because of his panicked, horrified tone.

Mindlessly, I steered Peyton toward the chairs in the distance. Glancing back, I overheard the agent explain, "Sir. You have a suspicious substance in your bag. I need you to remove the container and show me its contents."

Jamie watched anxiously as we disappeared around the corner. Turning to the security agent, he forced a smile, "If we could just step over here for a minute, I'll explain."

Understanding slammed into my brain and I staggered under its weight. Jamie would later tell me that his identification badge provided enough credibility and alleviated enough suspicion that the agent believed him and sympathetically spared him from having to open the brown box, and sparing Abby further indignity.

Our eyes locked as he joined us moments later in front of the escalator, "What happened?"

His tense smile could not hide the torture he had endured in convincing a stranger that the tiny powdery pile in the plain brown box composed what remained of his daughter. He nodded toward the escalator, "Nothing. Don't worry about it."

Once again, he suffered the moment alone. I bit down on my lip, fighting the sadness flooding my body. If I surrendered to it, I would crumble right there on the floor of the airport. Peyton's presence forced me to shove the pain deep into my soul. I hoped that in moments, the numbness would settle over me.

I stood, grasping the plastic blue chair, steadying myself. My chest tightened with every breath. My head throbbed. My eyes hurt. I was dizzy. Jamie stepped away, dragging the bags behind him. I followed, gripping Peyton's hand. My eyes were fixed on Jamie's suitcase.

The gate agent kindly allowed us to sit in business class for the long flight from Miami to San Francisco. Flying as non-revenue passengers, protocol required we sit in coach because of Peyton's age. The agent uncharacteristically ignored this rule with a wink. The bustle of Miami International and the irritating tone passengers often took with gate agents usually created a professional coldness. Peyton's smile must have melted her austerity.

When we boarded, Jamie took the bags and I busied myself strapping Peyton's car seat into the roomy seat. The last remnants of pregnancy hormones heightened my sense of smell and I gagged on the musty stale air and strong coffee brewing in the galley. I glanced at Jamie as he lifted our bags into the overhead compartment. I winced thinking of the little container of ashes, the remnants of my daughter, shoved into an overhead compartment. The thought broke my heart over and over throughout the excruciating flight.

That night, the three of us climbed into the big hotel bed, exhausted from the flight and the two-hour drive from San Francisco to Monterey. Peyton loved staying in hotels because we shared a bed. When she was a baby, we often let her fall asleep in bed with us. Our decision that she should learn to sleep on her own when she was a toddler ignited an intense battle that lasted for weeks. Many nights of crying and fighting tested my usually bottomless patience. Because of this, we no longer let her sleep with us, except in hotels.

She happily climbed into bed and curled up with Pooh. I fluffed the crisp, white sheet and let it float down over her, carrying its reassuring smell of bleach. She drifted to sleep quickly as I stroked her hair. I soon heard Jamie's rhythmic breathing as he, too, gave in to the fatigue. I shut off the television and the black hole that seemed to exist only in hotel rooms engulfed the room. I touched my eyes to see if they were open or closed. In the absence of sight or sound, my mind refused to stop spinning the images of the day. I pulled the cool sheet to my chin and rolled to my side. A sliver of moonlight suddenly poked through a crack in the curtain and rested on Jamie's suitcase. A solitary tear slid down my cheek and I closed my eyes.

In my dreams, I see our two girls.
Scrambling along the beach,
running in the waves,
creating sandcastles.
Singing, playing, dancing.
Sisters,
Friends.
At night, curled up together,
listening as I punctuate each word I read with effect.
Popsicles in the summer,
snowballs in the winter,
giant leaf piles in the fall.
Sisters.
Friends.
It is not to be.

16

Despite the late night, Peyton woke at 6:30, just like any other day. She snuggled in bed with Pooh watching Disney Channel while I drank coffee on the balcony. I hugged my knees and tucked a blanket under my feet, warding off the chilly breeze. I cupped the mug with both hands for warmth and watched the gray light of early morning disappear. Four years had passed since we'd last been in Monterey, but I had never forgotten its beauty. On our honeymoon, after spending four days in San Francisco, we drove to Carmel to spend two nights at the Highland Inn, an exquisite hotel overlooking the ocean off the Pacific Coast Highway. We anticipated stopping at Pebble Beach on the way and taking a quick drive along the Seventeen-Mile Drive. Our diversion changed our lives. We spent the entire afternoon stopping at each station along the Drive, soaking in its unique beauty. It is the most spectacular place on Earth. For this reason, we found ourselves in Monterey again.

Our day began with unassuming normalcy: pancakes at Denny's followed by an aimless drive around town. I asked Jamie to leave Abby's ashes in the hotel room because I didn't want them stashed in the trunk while we ate at a diner and drove around. Our mundane every day acts seemed to trivialize the gravity of the day. During breakfast, we decided to spend the morning at the Monterey Aquarium. I finished the cardboard pancakes in an attempt to calm the jitters caused by copious amounts of coffee. They sat like bricks in my stomach. Strangely, we were alone in the diner, which allowed us to tarry until Peyton grew impatient with boredom.

As Jamie maneuvered the maze of streets in downtown Monterey, the landmarks blurred by, my mind unable to assimilate them into my memory. These fleeting moments left no memories. We found the aquarium, looming over Monterey Bay with towering gates. Because we were early, we strolled along Cannery Row, peering out at the Bay as it awakened. The low tide pulled the sand into the Bay and the sea gulls searched for breakfast. Their screeching was accompanied only by the low roar of the water.

We soon returned to the aquarium, holding Peyton's hands and swinging her through the air, savoring her laughter and the illusive normalcy of the morning. As we passed people on the street, we met smiles and kind faces. In South Florida, eyes did not meet in public but looked off with imaginary urgency or preoccupation. For a moment, I considered whether somehow the universe was treating us kindly that day. I dismissed the thought, knowing that we were simply experiencing the nature of Californians.

At the aquarium, we chased Peyton as she ran from exhibit to exhibit unable to contain her excitement over seeing an octopus, sting rays, jelly fish, penguins, and a vast array of fish. Her tiny fingers curiously touched the glass, and she giggled as the fish darted away. What lay ahead crept into my mind. The sadness anchored my soul, dragging me away. But then Peyton's laugh, her joy, and her sweet little hand in mine pulled me back to the pleasure of the moment, giving me a sense of hope.

We discovered an amphitheater in the middle of the aquarium with massive stone steps and the sea as its stage. We huddled together. The air was crisp but heavy with salt. Breathing in, I could taste it. The sun warmed us and Peyton leaped down to the sea wall, dancing. A single rock jutted from the center of the Bay showcasing a sea lion sunbathing. Sea gulls circled, squawking at him, taunting him. We sat quietly, peacefully. The moment frozen. Finally, Jamie and I glanced knowingly at one another. We could no longer deliberate. The day was slipping away. We did not have the luxury of time to continue the façade of being just another family of tourists. Sadly, we turned our backs to the sea and climbed the stairs.

Peyton played on the hotel balcony as I stood guard over her, afraid to turn away from her for even a moment. Jamie busied himself in the room, flipping through hotel brochures, studying maps. We did not speak. We were lost. Knowing and not knowing what to do. We came to California to scatter our daughter's ashes. The moment loomed. My heart raced. I was not ready to go to Pebble Beach. I was not ready to let her go. Although what remained of her filled only a small brown box, to release its contents would be to release her forever. I was not ready.

Jamie broke the silence, suggesting that we have lunch, and I quickly agreed. This would grant more deliberation, more delay. We would drive towards Pebble Beach and stop somewhere along the way. Peyton took afternoon naps and we hoped that after lunch she would fall asleep as we rode to the sea. I knew that I was going to fall apart in Pebble Beach, no matter what strength I reserved or how much I fought. I knew that I could not pour Abby's ashes into the ocean and not crumble. I also did not want to be numb and unfeeling. I owed her my heart, my sorrow in that moment. To hold it in and not release it with her would be a betrayal.

Peyton and I stepped into the hallway and headed for the elevator. Seconds later, Jamie emerged from the room, the brown box in his hand. I shivered in pain. As the elevator doors opened and we stepped inside, I turned to him but avoided his eyes. The box held more than just ashes, it held the last physical presence of her. Once they were poured into the ocean, only her spirit and our broken dreams would remain. Jamie held the brown box in one hand and Peyton's hand in the other, tenderly clinging to his two girls. His face twisted as he, too, bore the weight of the moment. I prayed for strength and that my sanity would not be lost.

Peyton asked me to sit in the back seat with her. I glanced at Jamie and he nodded. I didn't want him to be alone in that front seat, but his eyes reassured me. Happily, I climbed in, welcoming the excuse to be close to her. I wanted to hold her hand, to touch her, to feel her life and her sweetness. Jamie put the brown box in the floor board of the front seat. Once again, he protected me.

As we drove through Monterey, the curtain of haze that typically blanketed the January Northern California sky lifted, forming a seamless canvas of sea and sky. Peyton and I watched the boats in the bay, weaving fanciful stories of their adventures. She searched the water for mermaids.

Abruptly, she turned to me, "Mommy, why is Baby Abby up in the sky?"

The suddenness of her question punched me. I could not help but begin to cry, unable to speak.

"Why, Mommy, why? Why is she up in the sky?" There was no sadness in her voice, only confusion as her little mind tried to comprehend. It was as if she knew why we were in California. Although she did not understand, she sensed our sorrow.

I laced my fingers with hers, "Remember when I told you that Baby Abby was very sick? Well, she was too sick to come home with us, so she went to live with God."

She jerked her hand away and crossed her arms, her voice full of indignation, "Why did she have to go live with God? I want her here."

I could not answer her question. I had no answer to that question. I had demanded one from God everyday, but He had ignored my pleas for understanding and peace. I cupped her chin then placed her cheek in my palm, "Me, too, baby. But she couldn't come home. I'm sorry. But remember that you can talk to her whenever you want."

She turned her face to the window, peering up at the sky, then raised her little hand and waved. She glanced back at me just as a tear escaped from behind my sunglasses, "Mommy, why are you crying?"

I smiled, my tattered heart soothed by her sweetness, "I'm just sad, baby. I miss Baby Abby."

"Me, too, Mommy." She reached over and placed her little hand on mine. Her love flowed through her fingertips into my heart. Bringing her had been the right decision. Her love, her innocent acceptance of what happened, pulled me from the brink. Jamie's strength allowed me to live each moment. Peyton saved my soul.

The pieces of my reality exist in the kaleidoscope that is my mind.
With each twist, my perception changes.
With each moment, the view becomes skewed.
What is real?
And what is the distortion created by my agony?
Beauty becomes horror,
Power becomes force,
Strength becomes violence,
Murmurs become thunder,
Vast becomes void,
Pain becomes normalcy.

17

Just outside of downtown, we stopped at a pizzeria along a side street. Strangely empty like the diner where we ate breakfast, we steered Peyton to a table abutting the windows. The air smelled of mildew and stale beer, but I knew it did not matter. I wouldn't taste the food anyway. I sat next to the window across from Peyton and watched as she scribbled on the paper placemat.

Jamie broke the uncomfortable silence, "I think what we're doing is the right thing."

I mulled the words over in my brain, trying to embrace their reality. His certainty comforted me because I could not find my own.

His looked down at the table, tracing an imaginary line around and around in circles, "This place is so special to us."

I stopped his fingers and held them in my hand, "Even if we had never been here, it would be perfect. It is the most beautiful place on Earth."

His eyes met mine and agreed.

After picking at the pizza, we climbed back into the car. Although I had tried to prepare myself the entire morning, knowing that the moment had arrived leveled me. The pain in my heart became physical and excruciating. My mind began spinning, my soul screaming at me, "I'm not ready. Not yet." The heaviness overwhelmed me and I didn't know if I could do what we'd planned. But it was time. We had only a few hours of daylight left.

Each mile, each moment closer to Pebble Beach, tugged harder on my composure. I felt my sanity slipping away. I hoped Peyton would soon fall asleep because I was falling apart. I breathed slowly, deliberately, trying to drive my tears down. I knew she would not understand and would be afraid. To see me cry was necessary, but to see me breakdown would change her. I bit my lip and took another breath. I no longer prayed. My prayers had been ignored. God had taken my daughter and abandoned me.

A kind face greeted us at the unassuming entrance gate. Its simplicity belied the grandeur of what lay ahead. He handed us a map and wished a good day to this family of tourists taking the Drive. Peyton asked where we were and where we were going.

Honestly, I answered, "For a drive."

Jamie and I had decided only on Pebble Beach. We had not discussed which part of Pebble Beach. The beach? The cypress forest? The overlook where the sea lions sunbathed? We both knew that when we felt it was right, we would know.

The map reminded me of the diversity of Pebble Beach. Scanning it, my eyes fell on the point along the Drive where the Lone Cypress stands. In the midst of the cypress forest, a small island juts out into the sea. On it sits a single cypress tree, which is named "The Lone Cypress." I thought it sounded like a good place for Abby. The Lone Cypress not only commands attention in its beauty and solitude, but it hovers over the sea, watching the sea otters play. I tucked the thought into the back of my mind, leaving it open for what we would find at the beginning of the Drive as we made our way along the beach.

After passing the Inn at Spanish Bay, the sea greeted us with its amazing beauty. I had forgotten the details: the rocks, the waves, the crispness of the air, and the sound of the sea crashing into the jagged shore. Magnificent. We lived only miles from the beach in Florida, but the Pacific Ocean is vastly different from the Atlantic. Our beach echoed the pace of Florida and its tourists on vacation. The waves slowly roll into the sand and gently pull it back out to sea. The sound is a low roar, a soothing purr.

In California, the ocean meets granite, with the result almost violent. The waves break hard against the rocks, splattering mist into the air. The current pulls the sea back harshly, scraping it over the reefs hovering under the surface. The roar is loud and the experience consuming.

Jamie cracked the window and the sea air rushed in, crisp but heavy. I smelled the salt and a roar filled the car. We decided to stop at Point Joe, which mistakenly appeared to be just a collection of rocks. Stepping up to their edge, we saw where the currents collide and the water is thrust into the air by an unseen force. Waves burst from all directions, churning. The sapphire sea is turbulent and powerful.

Through the eyes of my grief, my perception of the beach changed. While breathtakingly beautiful, it now seemed violent, not peaceful. Standing there, I knew we would not throw Abby into the raging sea.

We climbed back into the car and continued. We passed Bird Rock, which is a giant rock looming just offshore where shorebirds, harbor seals, and sea otters rest and play on its boulders. We stopped next at the tourist overlook that dangled over the beach where the sea lions sunbathed, thousands lying side by side or on top of one another. The young ones toddled out to the ocean, barking and climbing over one another. Peyton ran back and forth, calling to us, assuming the playfulness of the sea lions. But we stayed only a few minutes. Tourists crowded us and the sea lions created a painfully playful atmosphere. We dragged our unwilling little princess back to the car once again. It felt as though we were on vacation, not there to bury our child.

We drove quickly through the crowded cypress forest where the cars and tourists obtrusively lined the paths. Although we had not expected complete privacy, the volume of people distracted us. These strangers unknowingly intruded on our most private moment. We pressed on to the Lodge at Pebble Beach near the end of the Drive, needing a break and a chance to reflect on our cursory drive and where we should let Abby go.

After a deliberate stroll through the Lodge, we reluctantly slipped back into the car. Without speaking, we agreed to return to the Lone Cypress. I sat in front with Jamie, knowing he needed me. We needed to share the weight of the stone in our hearts. I had taken the easy way out, sitting with Peyton and holding her hand, forcing him to ride up front alone with Abby. After buckling Peyton in and explaining that Daddy needed my help driving, I opened the passenger door and sat down without looking. I immediately felt the brown box on my leg. I gasped, then held my breath, gathering my strength. Jamie glanced over at me and offered a weak smile. I reached my hand out to him and closed my eyes, trying to give him a little piece of my strength.

Turning back onto the winding road, I purposefully leaned my leg against the brown box. Making our final run through Pebble Beach, I desperately clung to these tiny pieces of her. By touching the brown box, I touched her. Even though I knew in my heart that she would forever be a part of me, she would soon be gone.

We again passed the Ghost Tree, which I had somehow missed on the way to the Lodge. With its trunk bleached white from exposure to the sea and the wind, it snarled at us. The passing cypress trees also changed before my eyes. What had once seemed beautiful now seemed dark and eerie. The bare knarled branches of the cypress trees became witches fingers clawing at the sky. I shut my eyes, searching for peace.

They opened when the car stopped. The parking area for the Lone Cypress was less crowded than before. Peyton, too excited and stimulated, refused to fall asleep. Jamie scooped her into his arms and we made our way to the path. Peyton clambered out of his grasp and hopped down the long wooden staircase leading to the overlook. We left Abby in the car and slowly descended the steps. Only a few people lingered nearby. When we reached the platform, we held Peyton's hands and stood at the railing.

Perched on a rock towering over the ocean, the Lone Cypress remained unchanged. Its prickly olive needles covered the top branches, leaving its trunk bare. Silhouetted against the afternoon sky and sea, its solitude was stark and melancholy. It connected with neither the forest nor the sea. Never to become one with either, it was forever alone.

The trees along the coastline, eroded and withered, had died. Their starved roots ripped open the rocks where they had perished, defeated by the sea. The rocks created sharp edges, causing the waves to crash violently. The sound was thunderous and intimidating. What had seemed magical and mystical four years before was now too sad, too lonely, and too violent. I knew we could not leave her there either.

Jamie's eyes expressed the same hopelessness I felt. Without speaking, we resolutely stepped away from the railing. I had failed to notice the young Chinese couple, accompanied by an elder. The old woman walked up to Peyton and smiled. She did not say, "Hi, what's your name?" or "Aren't you pretty" or any of the usual things. She simply looked at her tenderly and said, "Do you know what Heaven is?"

Peyton, unphased by this stranger, shook her head.

The old woman raised her hand to the sea, "This is it."

My mouth dropped open and I looked at Jamie, whose eyes were wide.

She nodded at us, then turned and walked back to her family.

She caused us to pause, reconsidering whether to scatter Abby's ashes at the Lone Cypress. After lingering for another half-hour, listening to the sea and watching Peyton play, Jamie broke our silence, "Well?"

Knowing what he asked, I shook my head. My heart ached with the thought of throwing her into the wind in this desolate place, "Can we go back to the beach?"

He sighed, relieved, and nodded.

As we turned to climb back up the stairs, she caught my eye: a single, playful sea otter swimming just under the point. Rolling and flapping in the waves, she stopped to swim over to a duck fighting against the current, trying to reach the rocks for safety. The little otter swam next to the duck, as if offering help, until the duck finally scrambled onto the rocks and shook the water from its wings. Then the otter disappeared under the sea.

As you slip through my fingers,
you do not go quietly.
My heart hears every word you should have spoken.
Every tear you should have cried.
Every song you should have sung.
Every giggle you should have squealed.
Every whispered secret.
Every scream in anger.
Every prayer.
Every laugh.
Every "I love you" that will never cross your lips.
I reach for you furiously,
desperately,
futility.
You leave me.
With a broken heart
and tiny footprints on my soul.

18

After driving back through the cypress forest, we once again emerged at the beach. Jamie slowed the car almost to a stop, "Honey? I'm waiting for you to tell me where to stop."

I could not answer him. I didn't know where to stop. My mind was incapable of such a decision. I assumed he would stop when he knew it was right. Whatever he decided would be right. I trusted in that. He searched my eyes for guidance. When none came, he continued driving. The minutes slowed as the end of our journey neared. The fog rolled in and the sun disappeared behind it. Peyton, still awake, sang softly in the backseat. Her happiness clutched tightly to the remnants of my sanity. Had she been asleep and silent, it would have left me.

I then remembered seeing a pedestrian path near China Rock. There had been a small patch of beach with a concrete pull-off, "Honey, there was a place near China Rock where we can stop. Why don't we pull in and figure out what we want to do instead of just driving?"

Happy to have input from me, he agreed.

We drove past Bird Rock and the area came into view. He looked at me and smiled. It was perfect. We had found the place. How had we passed it before without knowing? I suppose we had not been ready.

Jamie glanced over the roof of the car as he shut the door, "What should we say to Peyton?"

I knew he needed me to handle this, "I'm just going to tell her that we're going down to the water to find seashells. She loves doing that at home."

His voice dropped to a whisper, "But what will you tell her that we're doing?"

My heart knew the answer, "I'll tell her that we're sprinkling angel dust. We can't tell her what it is. She won't understand."

Although the brown box sat on the floor of the passenger side, I did not pick it up. Jamie walked around while I opened the back door and began fumbling with Peyton's car seat harness. I purposefully averted my eyes as I heard him open the box. A few seconds later, it closed. He emerged from behind the door with it.

We started towards the beach, the three of us holding hands. The pebbles quickly changed to boulders and moved under our feet. I worried that Peyton would fall, but she held tightly to our hands and climbed down easily, talking and singing incessantly. As we continued down the rocks, we saw an area to our left. Two massive collections of large boulders were divided by a small valley of sand and pebbles. We watched the waves break on the outer rocks, then gently slide into the valley, leaving tiny pebbles that glistened despite the fading sunlight. This was the place where we would bury our daughter.

Holding Peyton's hand, I reached down with the other and began picking up tiny headstones.

"Pey Pey? Why don't you look for rocks with Mommy? Pick beautiful ones and we'll take them back to Florida, okay?" I wanted her to be distracted and oblivious to us. She clambered around and quietly picked up stones, stopping to splash in the puddles.

Jamie wrapped his arm around me and pulled me to him. Tears filled my eyes and I felt sobs welling up from my soul. I clenched my teeth and slipped my arm around him. We stood silently, listening to the waves and watching as they slowly rolled into the valley. Then suddenly, strangely, a peace swept through me. I felt Abby's little footprints on my heart and knew she was with us.

Jamie opened the brown box and withdrew a silver cylinder. His hands shook as he opened the cylinder and pulled out a tiny clear bag. He held it out to me and I gently cradled it in my hands. I could not believe what I saw. It contained only a handful of gold and white flakes. This tiny bag of ashes was all that remained of my daughter, my beautiful, sweet Abby. I had held her in my arms. I had kissed her sweet lips, caressed her fingers, and touched her hands and her tiny eyelashes. Now nothing remained but a tiny pile of ash. I sucked in my breath. I could not contain my tears as they flowed down my cheeks. My heart ached and I felt as though it were happening all over again. I was falling into an abyss.

Then I heard Peyton singing nearby. I looked over and saw her innocently picking up stones and placing them in her pocket. I closed my eyes. I heard the wind, and in it, Abby's voice again. Again, she whispered Peyton's name. The sorrow in my heart disappeared and was replaced by an intense love for both of my girls.

Jamie opened the tiny bag and turned to me. Without thinking, I held out my hand. I wanted to hold her one last time before she left us forever. He poured some of her ashes into my hand and I cupped my palm, shielding them from the wind, and looked at them intently. Then, I gently touched them with my fingers.

I stepped away and searched the valley. A single rock jutted just above the stream where the waves slid in. I kissed my finger then placed it on her ashes as a final goodbye. I laid them on the rock where they glistened and waited. Within moments, the waves crashed against the outer rocks and a slow stream of water slid into the valley and over the rock where Abby's ashes waited. The tide created tiny dancing bubbles. The water then pulled back into the sea, taking Abby with it.

Jamie walked over to the rock with the tiny bag. As he poured what remained of her ashes onto her tombstone, I began to cry. A tearing pain ripped my heart. My sweet girl who had been alive inside of me, kicking and dancing, was now a small pile of ash lying on a rock, waiting for the sea. The water returned, washed over the rock, and Abby disappeared. Jamie stepped back to me and wrapped his arm around me again. Peyton, oblivious to what had just occurred, joined us, slipping her hand into mine. Time stood still as the three of us watched the waves slither in and out of the valley.

Jamie suddenly let go of our hands and ran back to the rock, "Honey, come here. There are still ashes on it!"

My heart jumped. She was not gone yet, "Really? Come take Peyton's hand, hurry, so I can look."

I quickly maneuvered the rocks and stepped into the stream. A few ashes remained on the rock. Again, I kissed my finger and placed it there. I solemnly stepped away and returned to Jamie and Peyton. I don't know how long we stood there staring at the rock. Abby's tombstone. Peyton, unaware but sensing something, stood with us quietly.

Jamie broke the silence, "What do you want to do with the box?"

I had not considered this, "I don't know. What do you think?"

He hesitated, looked around, and then decided, "We should leave it. We should leave all of it here."

He sounded so certain and peaceful. But I didn't want to just leave it lying on the beach, "Why don't we put it in the valley so the water can sweep it out to sea, too?"

He smiled, "Yeah. That sounds perfect."

He walked back to the rock and placed the brown box next to it. I held Peyton's hand and took mental pictures, never wanting to forget this place where we gave Abby back to God. This magnificent, peaceful place. This sacred and holy place. We three stood and watched as the water swept through the valley, nestled the box, and carried it out to sea. It slid behind the rocks and vanished.

Clutching Peyton's hands, Jamie and I climbed slowly back up the rocks, carrying our pebbles and the tiny bag. I opened my fist and smiled as I realized that there was a tiny bit of ash left in the corner of the bag; tiny pieces of her to keep. I had not wanted an urn to sit on a mantle, or on a shelf or in a mausoleum, but I cherished these tiny pieces to tuck away.

A sea of stones, marking the places of the dead.
Their bodies prostrate under the Earth.
Walking amongst them, I feel a tug at my spirit.
As if the dead are trying to claim it.
The air is heavy with the weight of souls. And grief.
This place does not evoke peace or joy.
My baby, my Abby, deserves a place that commands happiness.
A place of beauty and sweet remembrance. Not sorrow.
An immovable headstone created not by man,
But by God Himself.

19

There is a bench cemented into the earth at the top of the hill overlooking the valley between the boulders. I hadn't noticed it when we walked past it to climb down the rocks. It had been secured to the ground with permanency.

I knew it would be Abby's tombstone, "Honey, look at that bench."

Jamie glanced over and a knowing smile spread over his face.

I began walking towards the rental car, "Keep an eye on Pey. I'll be right back. Could you throw me the keys?"

My mind raced, wondering what I could use for a sharp edge. The car was littered with water bottles, maps, and Goldfish wrappers, but nothing sharp. I shut the door, settling on the keys to the rental car. As Peyton played in the sand, I sat down on the bench and looked out at the sea. The turbulence had calmed in the late afternoon. The water continued to move swiftly but rhythmically. The tiny pebbles along the shore glistened. The violent and lonely sense of death had been replaced with a sense of tranquility. The vastness of the sea no longer seemed foreboding but instead a timeless, limitless gateway.

Jamie sat next to me as I carved "ABBY" on the bench, "We can come back here whenever we want to be near her. We can sit on this bench, her bench, and touch her name and think of her."

He curled his arm around me, "Yeah."

I closed my eyes. The salty breeze brushed my face and filled my soul. I seared the memory into my mind. When I opened my eyes, I saw dozens of sea otters playing in the distance. It was as if they were waiting for Abby to come join them and play. Finally, I felt at peace. Jamie did too. I could sense it. In that moment, I felt closer to him than I've ever felt to another person. I closed my eyes again and made peace with God. I realized that He had not abandoned me, but had been with me through all of this horror, in the form of my sweet, little three-year-old angel.

My family was together, the four of us, in those final moments. I wanted to stay there forever. But the sun was setting and Peyton grew tired. As we stood to leave, I prayed with a grateful heart. Thankful that my incredible husband thought to go to Monterey. That he knew us so well to decide this, when I could not make any decisions.

Rather than driving back to the hotel, we detoured through downtown Carmel. Its quaint streets were lined with tiny shops and restaurants. The tourists strolled aimlessly, absorbing the unique beauty. We drove to the end of the block and parked in the beach lot. Peyton shrieked with happiness to be able to play a little longer in the sand. We arrived just in time for sunset. The sand at Carmel Beach is truly "sugar sand," so white and so soft.

The setting sun scarred the sky with a blazing red, orange, and yellow. I had never seen anything more beautiful. Beyond the sea were the cypress trees and the Seventeen Mile Drive. The only sounds were children laughing and the waves caressing the shore. As the brilliant sun melted into the sea, a few clouds dotted the sky. The fading sunlight shone through them creating beams that fell into the sea. It looked as if God had cracked open Heaven's door and spilled out its light.

Peyton ran back and forth, squealing and kicking up sand as she chased the waves. Jamie slipped his hand into mine and I leaned my head on his shoulder. Then, for a final time, I felt Abby's tiny footprints on my heart and heard her spirit whisper to me. A goodbye gently carried on the wind out to sea. As Peyton ran towards the waves, a solitary sea otter played offshore, spinning and flapping its arms. It swam towards us, poked its head up, and then disappeared under the waves.

One day, I will share with Peyton our day in Monterey. Never again will I look at a sea otter and not think of Abby. She will live forever in my heart. I miss her every moment.

Epilogue

Tyler Owen was born on April 18, 2004. One morning, when he was six months old, Peyton came into the nursery as I changed his diaper. She loved her baby brother, but had spoken often of Abby since his birth. She wanted a sister, too, she had told me. I never mentioned Abby. I didn't need to. Peyton remembered. When she drew pictures of the family, she included Abby as a little girl floating above the family.

As I snapped Tyler's onesie closed, Peyton asked, "Mommy, how old is Abby now?" She knew Abby lived in Heaven with God, but her mind could not fully understand. She believed Abby was growing up, too, and having birthdays.

"Well, baby, she's one now."

"Oh." Her smiled disappeared, "You mean she had her birthday and we didn't get to be with her."

I bit my lip when my tears started to sting my eyes, "She's always with us, baby. We may not have seen her on her birthday, but she was with us."

"Can we sing Happy Birthday to her, even though she already had her birthday?"

I could not help but kiss her in her innocent sweetness, "Of course."

She walked around me and patted Tyler on his head as she always did, "We're going to sing 'Happy Birthday' for your other big sister, Abby."

Tyler looked up at me. Not with the eyes of a baby, but with stillness. He stared into my eyes, not moving, as if he knew what we were saying.

I picked him up and kissed him, "Yeah, you know who we're talking about. You met her before you left Heaven, didn't you?" I cradled him in my arms, turned out the light, and followed Peyton's voice singing "Happy Birthday."

978-0-595-40603-6
0-595-40603-3